easy
pilates

cy
ime

A CONNECTIONS EDITION

This edition published in Great Britain in 2010 by
Connections Book Publishing Limited
St Chad's House, 148 King's Cross Road
London WC1X 9DH
www.connections-publishing.com

British Library Cataloguing-in-Publication data available on request.

ISBN 978-1-85906-311-8

1 3 5 7 9 10 8 6 4 2

Phototypeset in Meta using InDesign on Apple Macintosh
Printed in China

Contents

Introduction

In the first half of the twentieth century, Joseph Pilates – a gymnast and body builder, among other things – developed an innovative series of exercises by studying yoga and the movement of animals. His system – known today as 'Pilates' – has since been refined and updated, and is now widely practised around the world.

I have taught exercise to pregnant and postnatal women for many years, and Pilates is a safe and effective fitness system that can be easily adapted to suit the needs of both new and expectant mothers. Today's passive lifestyles mean that many of us are not as active as we should be, and pregnant women often use the excuse that pregnancy is a time for doing nothing by way of exercise. However, exercise can actually help relieve many of the discomforts of pregnancy (such as backache and swollen ankles), and keeping mobile reduces stiffness in the muscles and joints exacerbated by the body's centre of gravity moving forward during pregnancy.

A short sequence of exercise done regularly really benefits the body as it changes over the three trimesters. The exercises in this book are designed to keep the body strong throughout pregnancy and beyond, focusing especially on the arms, legs, back and pelvic floor, in preparation for an active labour, reducing the need for analgesia (and its effect on your baby and on your own recovery). Not only will your core strength, posture and body awareness improve, but you'll boost your immune system and enjoy increased levels of the 'feel-good factor', too. In addition, many of the exercises involve being on all fours, which encourages the baby to adopt the best birth position ('optimal foetal position', or OFP), thus promoting an easier, shorter labour.

How to use this book
As with any exercise regime, it's best if you practise regularly, building up your expertise over a period of time. I would suggest that you make a commitment to carry out the appropriate trimester sequence at least twice

a week, but ideally four times a week if you can, moving on to the next trimester when your pregnancy stage – or your body – dictates.

The book is divided into five exercise sections. Each corresponds to a specific period of pregnancy and, afterwards, the early postnatal months. The FIRST TRIMESTER sequence is designed for the first three months of pregnancy, and this section stands alone. The SECOND TRIMESTER sequence corresponds to four to six months, and the THIRD TRIMESTER seven to nine months. If you want a slightly longer session you can put the second and third trimesters together, although as your pregnancy becomes more advanced it's unlikely you'll want to exercise for as long as you may have done in the early stages, so you might like to stick to the THIRD TRIMESTER exercises only, during the final months or weeks.

The last two sections are for after the baby has been born. The EARLY DAYS sequence takes you from the birth up to approximately six to eight weeks post-birth, while EIGHT WEEKS PLUS is designed for eight weeks onwards, up to about five months after the birth. These two sections can be joined together for a full postnatal workout, but do be sure to wait until you've had your postnatal check-up with your doctor before you tag on the EIGHT WEEKS PLUS section. (Note: Following the birth many mothers need more time for healing to take place, particularly on the perineum, and even more so if there has been a tear or an episiotomy. Please allow the necessary healing time that is right for you.)

You will also find information on 'safe transition' – how to move safely from one position into another without placing undue strain on joints and muscles (see pages 56–7). It can be all too easy to move too quickly or twist awkwardly, causing damage that is easily avoidable. In addition, learning to breathe correctly is fundamental to effective Pilates practice, so make sure you read the information on pages 8–9 before beginning any of the exercises. There's also key information on the pelvic floor and posture on the pages that follow (see pages 9–13), so be sure to check that out, too.

All five exercise routines are featured on the handy quick-reference wall chart printed on the inside of the book jacket. Pin it up to aid your practice. The chart is colour-coded to match the book, so that you can easily cross-refer to the relevant page at any time.

Equipment
Stability balls, small balls, flexi-bands and blocks are used for some of the exercises to help you focus or to alter the intensity (or, in some cases, for comfort). These can be purchased inexpensively from sports shops or via the internet, but you could easily substitute a child's ball, folded towel and scarf for the small ball, block and flexi-band.

Many pregnant women find it worth investing in a stability ball, as this can be used during the birth: pelvic circles on the ball are quite soothing. Do make sure you get the right size for your height (if you have long legs, you might want to get the next size up): up to 5 ft 4 in (1.6 m), a 55 cm ball should suit; between 5 ft 4 in (1.6 m) and 5 ft 11 in (1.8 m), 65 cm; and over 5 ft 11 in (1.8 m), 75cm. When you sit on the ball, with your 'sit bones' right on top and your spine long, your thighs should slope gently down from hip to knee, so that your hips are slightly higher than your knees when sitting. If you don't have a stability ball, though, don't worry; simply omit the exercises that require one.

It is a good idea to invest in a non-slip exercise mat, if you don't already have one. Again, these are inexpensive, and will make the stability-ball work more stable.

Do what's right for you
Although the exercise sections have been divided into three trimesters, remember that everyone – and each pregnancy – is different. Some people suffer with nausea in the first trimester, while others feel fine right up to the final weeks. Expectant mothers are therefore encouraged to be responsible for themselves when exercising. Above all, listen to your body; stop an exercise immediately if you feel any pain; and take a break when you feel tired. (Around one in five women are affected by a condition called pelvic

girdle pain, or PGP. The majority of exercises in this book take PGP into consideration, but if you find that an exercise doesn't suit and produces pain in the pelvis, just leave it out and move on to the next one. For more information on PGP, visit www.pelvicpartnership.org.uk.)

Cautions are also included for some exercises, where specific warnings should be noted (for instance, if an exercise is unsuitable for use in another trimester). There are no abdominal curl exercises in this book, as it is not appropriate to work the top layer of abdominal muscles during pregnancy, but the deepest abdominal layer – the transversus – needs to remain strong to help support the back (*see also Breathing, overleaf*). Also, many pregnant women feel uncomfortable lying on their back after about sixteen to twenty weeks (if the baby lies on a blood vessel against the spine, it can restrict blood flow; this is why it is generally advisable to sleep on your side in mid- to late pregnancy), so none of the exercises for the second and third trimesters involve lying on your back. If you choose to do any exercises from the FIRST TRIMESTER section later on in your pregnancy, avoid those that are done in this position, or are contraindicated.

If you have any concerns about your health or ability to exercise, consult your doctor or healthcare professional before attempting the exercises in this book.

CAESAREAN SECTION If you have had a Caesarean section it is crucial that you don't lift anything heavy for at least the first two weeks, while the internal sutures heal. This includes car seats, prams, shopping, toddlers, and so on. Ask someone else to help with lifting during this time, or, if you have a toddler, ask them to climb onto your lap while you're sitting down. Most women who have had a Caesarean do not start formal exercise until at least eight weeks postnatally.

Breathing

Pilates breathing is integral to Pilates exercise. It may take a little time to master, but it's well worth the effort, as you will get more out of your Pilates practice. Pilates breathing is essentially lateral breathing, letting your rib cage expand out to the side and back as you breathe in, and breathing out through gently pursed lips, as though flickering a candle flame with your out-breath. Lateral breathing increases your oxygen uptake by about 25 per cent – very helpful while pregnant!

Always avoid holding your breath in any exercise. If in doubt, breathe out!

Try it: Stand or sit with your spine long. Breathe in through your nose (or mouth, if you prefer), letting your ribs expand out, then breathe out through your mouth, through pursed lips. Do this slowly, so you don't hyperventilate.

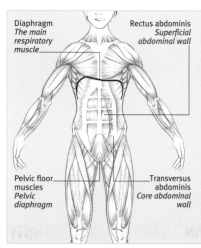

Diaphragm
The main respiratory muscle

Rectus abdominis
Superficial abdominal wall

Pelvic floor muscles
Pelvic diaphragm

Transversus abdominis
Core abdominal wall

CO-ACTIVATION OF TRANSVERSUS WITH THE DIAPHRAGM
The deep abdominal muscles (transversus) aid the diaphragm, so you will be using these muscles automatically when you breathe correctly. As you breathe in, feel the ribs expand out to the side, like gills; notice the muscles between each rib and the next rib flare laterally. As you breathe out, let these 'gills' sink and subside. Feel the deep abdominals drawn in smoothly and gently. Keep your shoulders relaxed throughout, and don't force inhalation or exhalation.

Effect of breathing on the pelvic floor

Breathing out as you do the hardest part of any exercise will help you to use the diaphragm, abdominal and pelvic floor muscles more effectively. As you breathe out, the diaphragm lifts upwards within the abdominal cavity, which means you can gently draw in the abdominals without putting extra pressure on the pelvic floor muscles (see below for more on the pelvic floor).

Breathing in this way also helps to tap into your autonomic nervous system, and this helps to release tension and produce feelings of relaxation. Some women also find that this deliberate focused out-breath through pursed lips helps them cope better with birth contractions.

Pelvic floor

The pelvic floor forms sling-shaped layers of muscles that are attached to the pubic bone at the front of the pelvis, the tailbone (coccyx) at the back, the 'sit bones' on each side at the base, and the walls of the pelvis. The sling has three openings: one at the front from the bladder (urethra), one in the middle from the birth canal (vagina) and one at the back from the bowel (rectum; *see diagram overleaf*).

What do the pelvic floor muscles do?

There are two types of muscle fibre in the pelvic floor: slow twitch muscle fibres and fast twitch muscle fibres. The slow twitch fibres have a constant tone in them (even when you're asleep) and work as a postural muscle. They also support your pelvic organs inside you, to help prevent prolapse, and help to keep urine inside your bladder until you find a suitable place to pass it. The fast twitch fibres contract strongly and quickly to control the bladder and prevent leakage of urine when you sneeze, cough, laugh or lift something heavy. They do this by pressing the urethra against the pubic bone, and the muscle fibres need to be strong to do this.

Why is the pelvic floor a focus during pregnancy?

These muscles are put under more pressure in pregnancy for two main reasons: the growth of the baby over the months in the uterus, and the

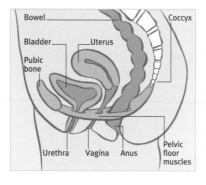

effect of the pregnancy hormone 'relaxin' on the ligaments in and around the pelvis, in preparation for the birth process through the birth canal.

This softening effect is not isolated to the pelvic region alone; relaxin loosens all the joints in the body, whether they are directly related to the birth or not. Some women even report joint laxity in the little finger! The effect of the hormone continues until approximately five months after the baby is born. This is why it is so important during pregnancy to treat your pelvis with respect and care, and to keep all your joints and muscles in good alignment, so reducing strain on the joints.

FINDING YOUR PELVIC FLOOR MUSCLES

- Sit on a firm chair, stool or block, in good posture. Tighten the ring of muscles around your back passage (anus), as though preventing a bowel movement or wind escaping. Lift the muscles up inside, hold for a second, and then relax slowly.
- Tighten the muscles around your back passage again, then take this feeling through to your front passages. Lift the back and front passages up inside, hold for a second, then relax them slowly.

When you tighten the pelvic floor muscles during an exercise, it is important to actually feel the release of the muscles again, as you return the pelvic floor to the start position. Never perform pelvic floor exercises while you are passing urine, as this causes a risk of developing a urine infection (during pregnancy this risk increases, if the exercise is not done correctly).

Exercising the muscles

Slow twitch The slow twitch muscles need to be recruited smoothly and gently. Their strength needs to be built up gradually over a period of weeks. As with all exercise regimes, you need to determine where you are starting from, so that you can measure progress and be motivated by improvement.

To determine your 'starting block':

- Tighten your pelvic floor muscles smoothly and gently, as described above. Hold for as many seconds as you can (up to a maximum of ten seconds). Relax the contraction and rest for four seconds. How long could you hold the contraction for? Note down how many seconds.
- Now, repeat the muscle contraction gently and smoothly. Tighten, hold for the number of seconds just noted, and relax, repeating this as many times as you can (up to ten repetitions). How many times could you repeat the contraction? Note down how many repetitions.

So, this becomes your 'starting block' – the number of seconds you can hold and how many repetitions (up to ten) you can do (for example, two seconds with four repetitions). You won't be able to hold for long at first, but do continue to practise, as the muscles will get stronger.

Fast twitch These muscles need to be able to react strongly and quickly, preventing leakage when you squeeze them tightly. See how many quick and strong contractions you can do, and note down the number of repetitions. Aim to make the last repetition as strong as the first.

Repeat a balance of the slow and fast muscle contractions between three and six times a day. For optimum pelvic floor health, make this a habit for life, not just for the three to four months retraining following the pregnancy and birth!

If there is weakness in the pelvic floor muscles, you may be more aware of an increased leakage of urine during the second and third trimesters. In the third trimester the increased weight of the baby also makes it harder to be aware of the pelvic floor working in a standing or sitting position, so it's a good idea to do the exercises while lying on your side, to get a good contraction of the muscles. It is important you continue to practise these pelvic floor exercises throughout your pregnancy.

Pelvic floor and transversus

The deep abdominal (transversus) muscles and the pelvic floor co-contract, which means that whenever you recruit one, the other will be working as well. However, the way the muscles work together is affected during pregnancy, so it's important to work these muscle groups separately. Also, research is clear that to strengthen the pelvic floor you need to exercise both fast twitch and slow twitch muscle fibres regularly over a period of months.

Make sure you draw in the transversus smoothly and gently; if you strongly activate the rectus abdominus (the top layer of the abdominals), then intra-abdominal pressure rises and forces the pelvic floor muscles downwards. This means even more pressure on the pelvic floor; not what is needed!

Birth and beyond

When preparing for the birth you also need to learn how to relax the pelvic floor muscles, ready for the baby's head crowning. Consider getting in touch with a birth-preparation organization, to find out more about the birth process and how you can help yourself through good information and knowledge of the choices in childbirth.

Once your baby is born you will need to re-educate both types of pelvic floor muscle fibre. You can start pelvic floor exercises again as soon as you can pass urine normally (*see also page 94*). At this point, your 'starting block' will need to be reassessed, as well as renewed motivation found, especially when there are so many other things to attend to with the arrival of your baby. But don't give up!

Posture

Correct posture is essential to help your body cope well with the changes that occur during pregnancy. As your baby grows you will be carrying extra weight, and this pulls your centre of gravity forward – often resulting in an over-arching of the lower back, and subsequent pain. When the body is misaligned it has to work harder to maintain an upright stance, and muscles tire easily when out of alignment. Many of the exercises in this book are thus designed to rebuild strength and shape where muscles have weakened or tightened.

Standing and sitting in good posture each day will help alleviate these aches and pains and aid correct recruitment of the pelvic floor muscles. Try to be aware of your posture, and run through a posture check at least once a day.

STANDING POSTURE CHECK
- Stand with your feet hip-width apart, with your weight evenly distributed and your arms resting at your sides.
- Check that your knees are soft (not locked!) and in line with your toes.
- Lift your pubic bone slightly, towards your navel, lengthening your lower back and dropping your tailbone down more.
- Feel the deep abdominals (transversus) draw in smoothly and gently.
- Relax your shoulders and open the front of your shoulders a little.
- Lift up through your spine to create extra space around your ribs.
- Look straight ahead, allowing your chin to be parallel with the floor.
- Breathe in through your nose and out through softly pursed lips.

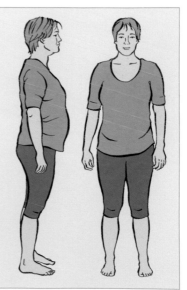

first trimester

This exercise sequence is designed for the first three months of pregnancy.

Always stop an exercise immediately if you feel any pain (stop and rest, and/or skip the exercise and move on to the next one), and be sure to note any specific cautions that are listed.

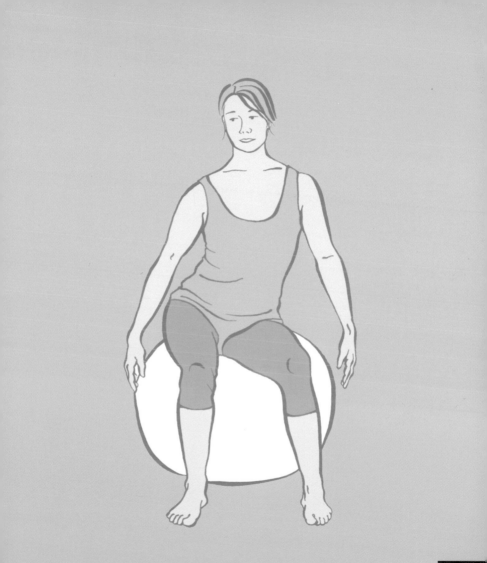

❶ Shoulder mobility

Improves shoulder mobility • Eases tension in the upper back • Helps stabilize the shoulder blades and improve upper back posture

Shoulder blade stability

Lie on the mat with your knees bent and feet flat on the floor, hip-width apart. Without letting your shoulders creep up towards your ears, float your hands up above your chest (the small ball is optional). Breathing in, stretch your fingers towards the ceiling, allowing your shoulder blades to slide around towards your arms, then breathe out and draw the sides of your ribs down (the serratus anterior muscles), and feel your shoulder blades draw down and flatten on your back.

Repeat five to eight times.

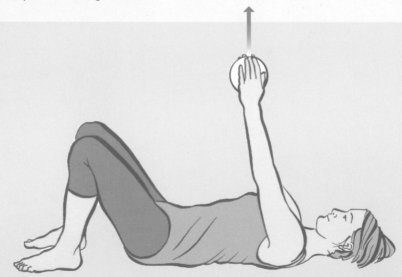

Shoulder rolls

1 Sit tall on a block or folded towel, with your legs crossed or comfortably bent in front of you. Feel your shoulders relaxed down your back and your abdominals working to hold your body quite upright.

2 Breathe in. As you breathe out, draw your shoulders up, over the top and down your back, releasing them down, away from your ears.

Repeat five to eight times.

TIP Use your side and back ribs to draw the shoulder blades down.

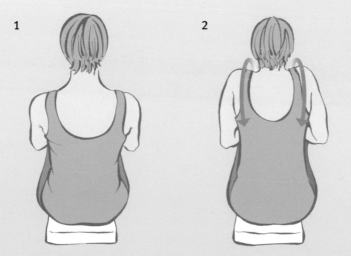

❷ Hip rolls

Mobilizes the spine • Works the abdominal group of muscles (assisted by buttocks and hamstrings)

Caution: This exercise does not suit everyone in early pregnancy. Suitable for the first trimester and postnatal period only; do not perform this exercise beyond sixteen to twenty weeks.

Lie on a mat or firm flat surface with your knees bent and feet flat on the floor, hip-width apart, with your lower back in a natural, comfortable shape (called 'neutral' spine). Your arms should be relaxed at your sides.

1 Breathe in to prepare and, as you breathe out, draw your abdominals in smoothly and gently and draw your ribs down towards your pelvis,

1

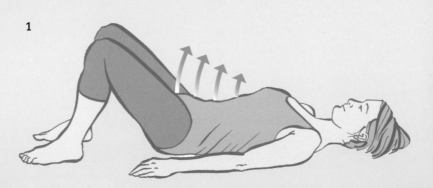

tipping your pelvis up towards your ribs (this position is often called 'imprint'). Moving on your next out-breath, pick up your tailbone and lift your spine off the mat each vertebra in turn. Continue until your spine is long and lifted into a diagonal line from the shoulders through the hips, and up to your knees.

2 Breathe in here, without lifting any higher, and feel long through the body. Then breathe out and reverse the process, returning to the floor, vertebra by vertebra, until the tailbone is back on the floor again.

Repeat five to eight times.

TIP Use the abdominals to start and continue the movement in both directions, feeling the lower back opening as you scoop in with the rectus abdominus muscle. Your neck and shoulders should remain relaxed.

2

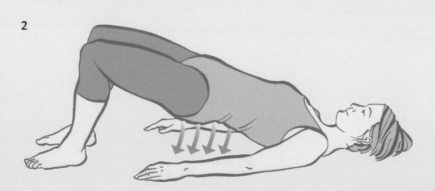

❸ Cat arch

Improves and maintains abdominal group of muscles • Helps keep the spine flexible

Caution: If you experience pain in your lower back, knees or wrists, try this exercise with a stability ball, as used in the second trimester (*see page 60*).

1 Kneel on all fours, with your hands under your shoulders and your knees under your hips. Keep your whole back in line, like a flat table, and the back of your neck long, with your shoulders released down your back. Keep your abdominal muscles activated to prevent the lower back from sagging.

1

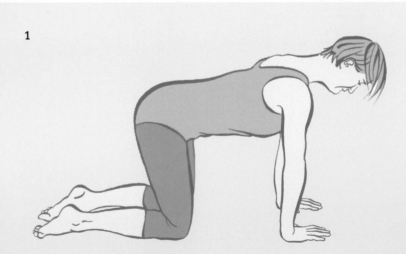

2 Breathe in to prepare and, as you breathe out, draw the abdominals in gently and smoothly, then curl under with your tailbone and start to tighten your abdominal 'zip' muscles (rectus abdominus) quite strongly, curling your spine towards the ceiling, each vertebra in turn. Lastly, feel your neck release to allow you to look through to your knees. Feel the whole abdominal group of muscles initiating the movement and working, and the lower back opening up.

Breathe in to maintain, then, as you breathe out, reverse the exercise, starting with the pelvis, taking care not to let the lower back sag as you return to the start position.

Repeat five to eight times.

TIP Try to keep your shoulder blades released, sliding down the spine.

2

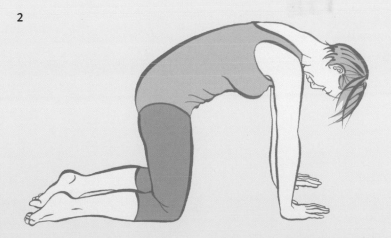

❹ Single-leg circles

Strengthens abdominal muscles • Increases flexibility of the hips

Caution: If you experience any pain in the lower back, bend the straight leg at the knee, with the sole of your foot flat on the mat.

1 Lying on your back, wrap a flexi-band or scarf around your right leg and bring it into 'table top' position (knee directly above the hip, and shin parallel with the floor). Cross the band once in front of the right thigh and take hold of either side, with the band just tight enough to give your leg some support. Allow your left leg to lie long along the mat, either bent or straight, depending on how your lower back feels.

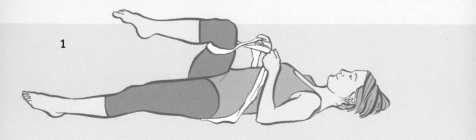

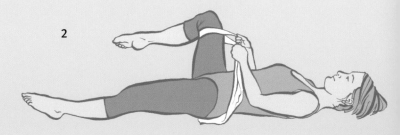

2 Breathe in to prepare, and stabilize the pelvis by drawing the deep abdominals in. As you breathe out, allow your right leg to go out to the side of your body.

3 Draw the leg down, away from the hip, and circle it across the body and back to the start position in 'table top'.

Repeat five to eight times, and then repeat with left leg.

TIP Keep the pelvis level and still, especially when your knee moves out beyond the side of the body. Try to recruit the deep abdominal muscles smoothly and gently throughout, and use them to keep the body quite still while the leg circles from the hip.

3

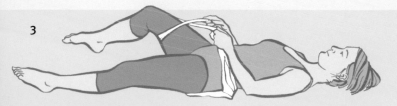

ALTERNATIVE
If you can keep the pelvis level and still, try it without a flexi-band, but bend your other leg at the knee, with your foot flat on the floor. This keeps the lower back safer.

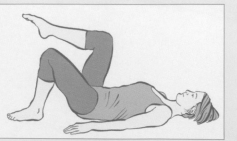

⑤ Spinal rotation

Maintains and increases spinal mobility • Works abdominal and postural muscles • Helps maintain front-of-shoulder 'openness', which commonly tightens during pregnancy

Sit cross-legged on a block, folded towel or directly on the mat, keeping the spine long and lifted. Gently draw up the pelvic floor muscles.

1 Hold a ball out in front of you at shoulder level, and relax your shoulders. (The ball is just for emphasis, so if you don't have one, just stretch your arms out.) Now breathe in as you bend the left elbow, bringing the ball to your underarm. Keep the fingers of your right arm stretching out in front of you.

1

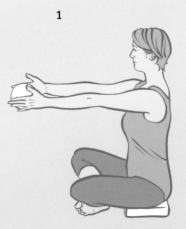

2 Breathe out and take the arm and ball behind you, twisting through the spine. Then breathe in and bring the ball back to the underarm, breathing out again to bring the hand and ball back to the start position in front of you, alongside the right hand.

Now rotate to the right. Take the ball in the right hand, breathe in to bend the right elbow, bringing the ball to the underarm, and breathe out to twist and take the ball behind you. Return as for the left hand.

Repeat each side five to eight times.

TIP Keep the fingers of the front arm stretching long as you twist round. The shoulders should remain relaxed and the spine long and lifted up to the ceiling throughout. Fix the hips and keep your weight firmly on both sit bones, to ensure rotation occurs in the mid not lower back.

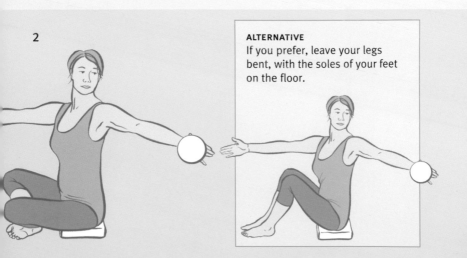

2

ALTERNATIVE
If you prefer, leave your legs bent, with the soles of your feet on the floor.

❻ Front-of-shoulder stretch

Stretches the chest and front of shoulders • Increases front-of-shoulder 'openness', which commonly tightens during pregnancy

Sit comfortably on a block, folded towel or directly on the mat, with your legs bent and feet flat on the floor (alternatively, sit with your legs crossed if you prefer). Place your fingertips behind you on the mat, to help keep your spine lifted and long, but don't lean back on your hands.

1 Breathe in to prepare and, as you breathe out, open the front of the shoulders, feeling the shoulder blades easing down your back.

1

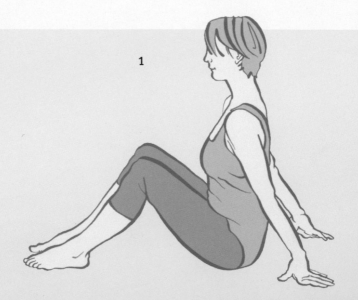

2 Feel a lovely stretch across the front of the shoulders and into the chest. Breathe in to maintain, then breathe out to release back to the start position.

Repeat three to five times.

TIP Keep your spine long and lifted throughout, and gently draw in the pelvic floor muscles.

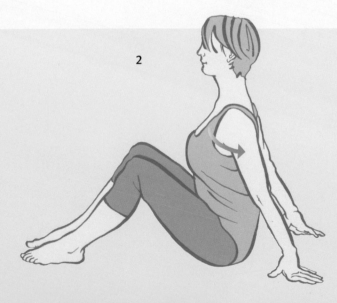

2

⑦ Single-leg stretch

Works the abdominal muscles

Caution: Suitable for first trimester and postnatal mothers only.

Lie on your back with your knees bent, with your shoulders relaxed and shoulder blades flat on the mat. Hold a small ball between your hands to help keep them in alignment. Bring your arms up to the ceiling above your chest, keeping the front of the shoulders open and the blades relaxed.

1   Breathe in to prepare and, as you breathe out, draw in your deep abdominal muscles, smoothly and gently, as you draw your ribs down towards your hips. Feel your lower back slightly imprinting. Allow your arms to move over your head towards the wall behind.

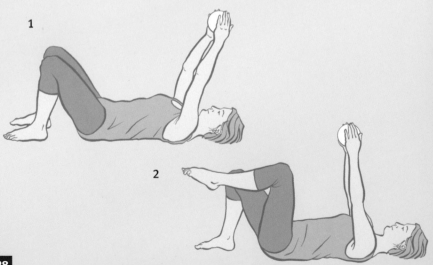

2 Bring your left leg up into the 'table top' position, with your hands above your shoulders, as before.

3 Breathe in to prepare and, as you breathe out, straighten the left knee, keeping the left thigh in line with the right thigh. Feel the left leg stretched long. As you straighten your leg, allow your arms to move over your head again, as in step 1, but this time making sure you keep the lower back drawn down into the mat a little more, as the intensity is higher here.

Repeat three to five times with the left leg, and then repeat the same number of times with the right leg.

TIP Feel your abdominals working and draw your lower back into the mat (imprinting) to avoid arching it.

3

⑧ Abdominal draw-in

Works all the postural muscles, including the abdominal muscles and pelvic floor

Sit on the stability ball, with your sit bones right on top of the ball and your feet hip-width apart, and feel your spine long and lifted. Bring your arms up to shoulder level in front of you, and try to keep your shoulders relaxed throughout. If you're having difficulty maintaining your balance, take your feet a little wider to make your start position more stable.

1   Breathe in to prepare and, as you breathe out, draw in the deep abdominal and pelvic floor muscles smoothly and gently. Breathe in to release. Repeat three to five times.

1

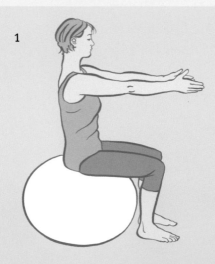

2 Next, if it feels OK to you, breathe in to prepare and, as you breathe out, draw in the deep abdominal and pelvic floor muscles again, and then lift your right foot about 5 cm (2 in) off the mat. Breathe in to return to the mat, then repeat with the left foot. Repeat three to five times with each leg.

TIP Keep the spine long and lifted as you work, helped by your abdominal muscles. Keep your sit bones on top of the ball, and try not to lean back as you lift your foot. Your shoulders should remain relaxed and the blades low down your spine throughout – don't hunch up.

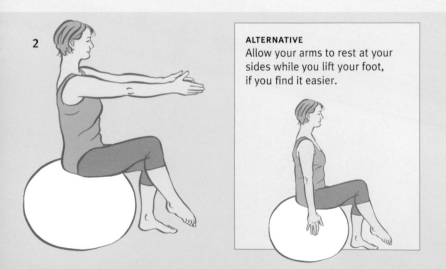

2

ALTERNATIVE
Allow your arms to rest at your sides while you lift your foot, if you find it easier.

⑨ Leg strengthener

*Works all the postural muscles, including the abdominal muscles and
pelvic floor • Works thigh muscles*

Sit on the stability ball, with your sit bones right on top of the ball and
your arms relaxed by your sides. Feel the spine long and lifted.

1   Breathe in to prepare and, as you breathe out, draw in the deep
    abdominal and pelvic floor muscles smoothly and gently.

2   Breathe in to maintain and, as you breathe out, straighten your right
    leg. Release back to the starting position as you breathe in again.

Repeat five to eight times, and then repeat with the left leg. You can
now move on to add scissor arms in the next step.

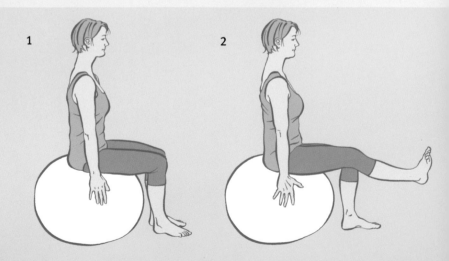

3 Bring both arms up to shoulder level out in front of you, keeping your spine long and your shoulders relaxed down. Breathe in to prepare and, as you breathe out, draw in the deep abdominal and pelvic floor muscles. Breathe in to maintain, but this time, as you breathe out and straighten your right leg, lift your left arm up, fingers towards the ceiling, keeping the arm fairly straight. Your other arm should remain at shoulder level. Breathe in to release your arm and leg back to the starting position, then repeat with your left leg and right arm.

Repeat five to eight times.

TIP Keep your shoulders relaxed throughout and feel the abdominals working to keep you upright and still on the ball.

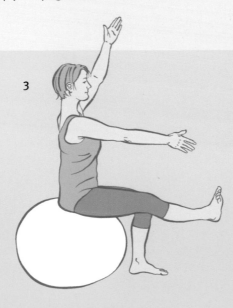

3

⑩ Side stretch

Works the abdominal muscles • Stretches the side of the body

Sit on the stability ball, with your sit bones right on top of the ball, and draw in your deep abdominal muscles. Leave your arms relaxed at your sides.

1 Breathe in to prepare and, as you breathe out, draw in the deep abdominal and pelvic floor muscles smoothly and gently. Then breathe in to bring your left arm up to the ceiling.

1

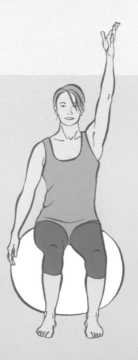

2 As you breathe out, lengthen your left side, lifting out of the left hip a little, allowing your left hand to come over your head as far as feels comfortable, while your pelvis remains stable on the ball. Breathe in to release back to the start position, but maintain the feeling of lift through the sit bones to help keep your spine long. Then repeat with the right arm, to stretch your right side.

Repeat three to five times.

TIP Try to keep the shoulders relaxed and shoulder blades down your back throughout, even though you are moving your arms.

2

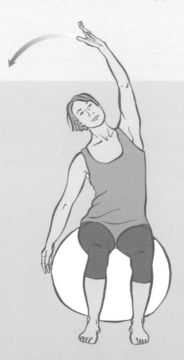

⑪ Arm strengthener

Helps maintain and improve arm-muscle strength (ready for the birth and caring for your baby) • Works the postural muscles

1 Sit on the stability ball, your spine long and lifted. Take the flexi-band round your back, level with your bra strap, bringing it under your arms and holding either end in each hand. Hold the band just tight enough to feel it slightly taut. Breathe in to prepare and, as you breathe out, draw in the deep abdominal and pelvic floor muscles smoothly and gently.

2 Breathe in again and, as you breathe out, bring your arms out in front of you in an 'A'-shape, feeling the arm and shoulder muscles working against the tension of the band. Breathe in to release the arms.

Repeat five to eight times.

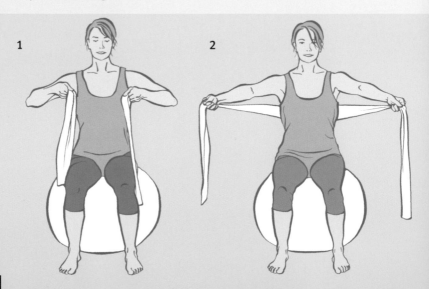

⑫ Pelvic circles

Helps ease out tension in the lower back • Lovely exercise to keep the pelvis moving during labour!

Sit on the stability ball, with your sit bones right on top of the ball, and feel the spine long and lifted. Think of the base of your pelvis as the four points of the compass – north, east, south and west.

Keep breathing easily as you allow your pelvis to start at north (the pubic bone), and rotate the pelvis round to the east (the right sit bone), then round to the south (the tailbone) and on to the west (the left sit bone). Then reverse and circle round the other way.

Feel the pelvis rotating and enjoy the loosening feeling through your lower back. Repeat five to eight times in each direction.

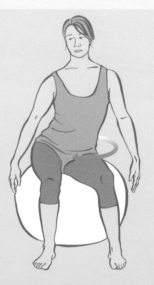

⓭ Leg pull

Helps maintain and improve shoulder blade stability, pelvis and lower back strength, and abdominals • Strengthens arms

Kneel on a mat on all fours, with your hands under your shoulders and your knees and feet together. Tuck your toes under, so that you are ready to come onto the balls of your feet.

1 Activate your deep abdominals and pelvic floor, and feel your ribs drawn down just a little towards your pubic bone. This helps to maintain the lower back in neutral (in other words, not over-dipped).

1

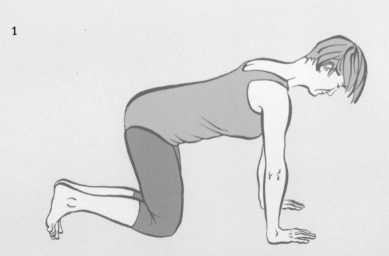

2 Keeping your shoulders drawn down and your abdominals working, breathe in to prepare and, as you breathe out, squeeze your knees together and your ankles together, and lift your knees 5 cm (2 in) off the floor – no more than that. This brings you up onto the toes and balls your feet. Breathe in to return your knees to the floor.

To develop more strength as you complete the repetitions, try to stay lifted for several in- and out-breaths.

Repeat five to eight times.

TIP Keep your spine long, shoulders stabilized, hips level and abdominals smoothly drawn in, despite your knees lifting.

2

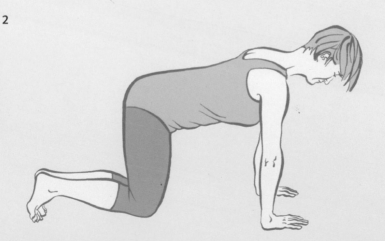

⑭ Press-ups

Helps strengthen the arm and chest muscles, ready for lifting and carrying your baby

Kneel on a mat on all fours, with your hands wider than your shoulders and your knees under your hips, feet relaxed and in line with your hips.

1 Activate your deep abdominals and feel your ribs drawn down just a little towards your pubic bone. As in the previous exercise, this helps to maintain the lower back in neutral (not over-dipped).

1

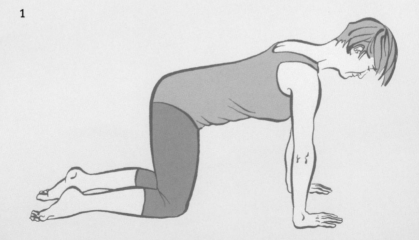

2 Keeping your shoulders drawn down and your abdominals working, breathe in with three little sniffs, as you bend your elbows back towards your knees, allowing your chest to come down towards the floor between your hands. Breathe out to push back up to the start position. Feel your arms and chest working throughout.

Repeat five to eight times.

TIP Try to keep your lower back supported and your shoulders and shoulder blades down your back, using your side ribs.

2

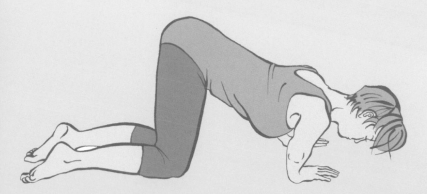

⓯ Spinal rotation (side)

Helps maintain spinal rotational mobility

Caution: If you experience any pain, particularly in the lower back, reduce the range of movement in the arm and torso.

1 Lie on your left side, with a block or folded towel under your head. Bring your knees up level with your hips (into a side-lying 'table top') and allow both arms to lie out in front of you, but with your shoulder blades flattened and drawn down your back, and your lower back in 'neutral'.

2 Breathe in and lift your right arm up to the ceiling.

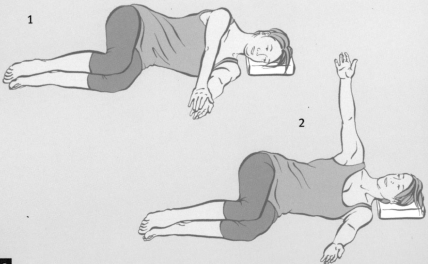

3 As you breathe out, open the front of the shoulder and take your right arm behind you, just as far as feels good. Allow your eyes to follow your right thumbnail as the arm goes behind you. Breathe in to maintain, and feel the stretch from one set of fingertips to the other, across the chest and front of your right shoulder.

Breathe out as you draw in the deep abdominals smoothly and gently, feeling your right ribs drawing down towards your pubic bone, and using these muscles to bring your right arm back to the start position.

Repeat five to eight times, then turn over and repeat with the left arm.

TIP Keep your knees heavy and in the same place throughout to ensure rotation is in the mid back, creating the return arm movement with the abdominal muscles.

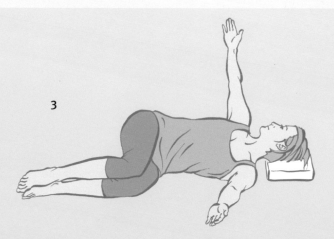

3

⑯ Side kick

Helps stretch and tone hamstrings and buttocks • Strengthens the abdominal muscles

Lie on your left side with your body near the back of the mat, with a folded towel or flat cushion between your arm and your head. Allow your legs to be straight, with your ankles near the front of the mat, so that there is approximately a 160-degree angle at the front of the hips. Feel your waist long on both sides of the body throughout the exercise.

1 Lift your right leg to hip height, keeping your knee straight and your ankle flexed.

1

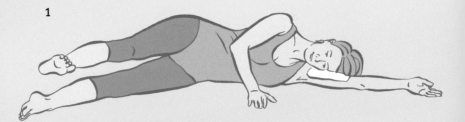

2 Breathe in, bringing the leg forward just as far as feels comfortable, stretching the back of the thigh a little. Avoid rolling off the supporting hip as the leg comes forward, keeping the leg at hip height.

3 As you breathe out, point the toe and bring the leg back to be in line with your body (remember that the lower leg is at a slight angle to the body), feeling the buttock working.

Repeat five to eight times, then turn over carefully and repeat on the other side.

TIP Use your lower leg to help you stay balanced by tightening the inner thigh and pressing the foot against the floor. Make sure you keep your top leg at the same height throughout; this strengthens the deep transversus, which works to keep the pelvis still as you bring your leg forward.

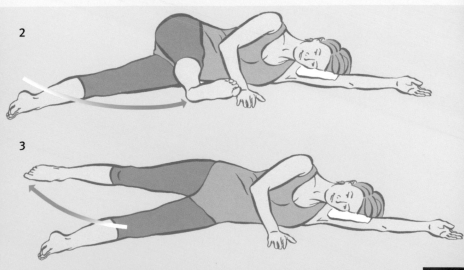

⑰ Side leg lift

Improves and maintains buttock strength (particularly helpful for walking later in pregnancy) • Helps with blood and lymph circulation in the legs and helps prevent/relieve swollen ankles • Helps strengthen the abdominal core muscles

Lie on your left side with your body and legs in line, and your shoulders and hips each 'stacked' one above the other. Bend your left (lower) ankle to help you balance, and place your right (upper) hand on the mat in front of your body, to help stabilize you.

1   As you breathe in, draw in your abdominal and pelvic floor muscles, then point your toes and lift your upper leg to hip height only, keeping the knee facing the front and stretching long through the leg.

1

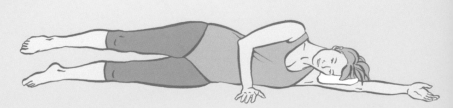

2 Breathe out, flexing the ankle, and feel a stretch through your heel as you bring your leg back down to the start position.

Repeat five to eight times, then roll over carefully onto your right side, and repeat with the left leg.

TIP Feel the waist staying long on both sides of the body, and feel stretched through the whole body as you work.

This exercise can also be done in the second and third trimesters, but it's a good idea to support your abdomen (and the growing baby) with a folded towel, as you should find this more comfortable.

2

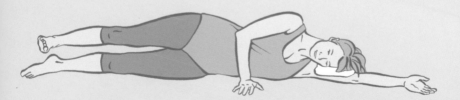

⑱ Side bend

Maintains and strengthens arm muscles (ready for lifting and carrying your baby) • Stretches the sides of the body • Keeps the spine flexible • Strengthens abdominals to support lower back

Caution: If you experience knee discomfort, do a seated side stretch, as used in the third trimester (*see page 84*).

Sit on your left side with your legs tucked up and slightly behind, out to the right, knees bent and legs and feet together. Place your left hand flat on the mat under your shoulder, with your arm straight and slightly out to the side.

1

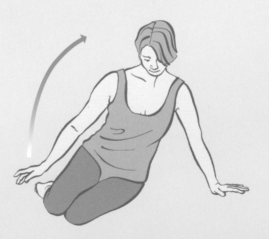

1 Breathe in to lift your right arm up to the ceiling, lifting your hips and body off the mat, transferring most of your weight onto your left knee and shin.

2 Breathe out and stretch your right hand over your head. Feel a stretch through the length of the right side of the body. Breathe in and lower back down to the start position, maintaining control.

Repeat three to five times, then carefully change over to sit on your right side, and repeat with the left arm.

TIP Try to feel the abdominal muscles and pelvic floor working. Avoid leaning forward – bend directly to the side.

2

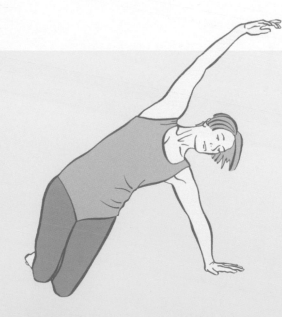

⑲ Saw

Stretches the hamstrings • Rotates the spine • Strengthens the postural muscles

Caution: This exercise gets progressively more uncomfortable as the pregnancy develops, so you may find it unsuitable in the second and third trimesters, as the baby gets bigger in utero.

Sit on a block or folded towel, if needed, with your right leg stretched out in front of you and the left leg bent and out to the side a little, with your foot flat on the floor.

1 Lift your spine long, towards the ceiling, and turn towards your right leg, bringing your arms up in readiness for the next step.

1

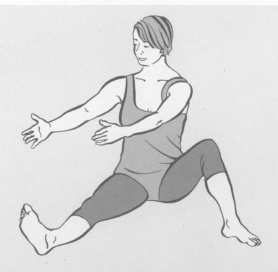

2 As you breathe out, reach your arms out over your straight leg, with your body following, and ease into a stretch for the hamstring (the muscles from the back of the knee to the sit bone). Feel a pleasant twist in the body as you lengthen your spine. Breathe in to return, but keeping the twist until you are upright again.

Repeat three to five times. Carefully change legs and turn to repeat to the other side.

TIP Feel a pleasant rotation of the spine as you work. Lengthen out of the hips as you stretch over the leg.

2

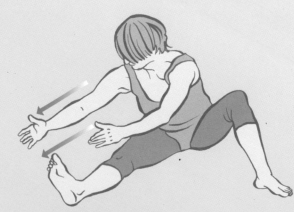

㉒ Shoulder opener

Lengthens the chest muscles and improves front-of-shoulder 'openness'.

1 Standing in good posture, keeping the spine long, gently clasp your hands behind you, noting which thumb is on top in the clasp.

2 Breathe in to prepare and, as you breathe out, gently draw in the deep abdominals and lift your hands up behind you, keeping your elbows soft, until you feel a good stretch across the chest and front of the shoulders. Keep your abdominals working, to ensure that your lower back doesn't over-arch. Keep breathing and hold the stretch for eight to ten seconds.

Release, change your clasp so that the other thumb is on top, and repeat.

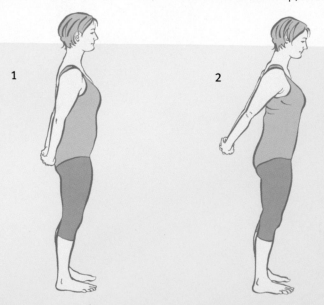

1

2

㉑ Adductor stretch

Lengthens the inner thigh muscles

Caution: If you feel pain in the pubic bone, stop immediately.

Sit on the mat with the soles of your feet together, and let your knees open to the sides. Place your fingers on the mat behind you.

Breathe in to prepare and, as you breathe out, gently ease your knees outwards until you feel a stretch on both the inner thighs (the muscles from the groin to the inner side of the kneecap). Try to draw in the deep abdominals, and keep the spine long and lifted.

Hold for eight to ten seconds, and release. Repeat if you wish.

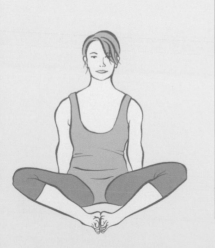

ALTERNATIVE
Some people need to hold their feet and lean forward to find this inner-thigh stretch. Try it out and see what suits you.

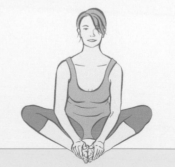

second trimester

This exercise sequence is designed for months four to six of your pregnancy. For a slightly longer practice session, you can join the second and third trimester sequences together.

Always stop an exercise immediately if you feel any pain (stop and rest, and/or skip the exercise and move on to the next one), and be sure to note any specific cautions that are listed.

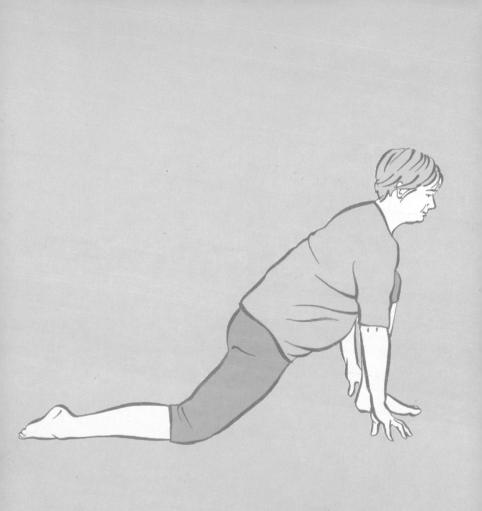

Safe transition

Following these simple steps will help you keep your body aligned more safely as you transfer from one position to another – especially important as your pregnancy advances – minimizing the chance of any damage to joints and the vulnerable abdominal muscles. Get into good 'safe transition' habits now and stick to them, as they are essential to abdominal recovery after the baby is born.

1 ▶ When lying on your side, place a folded towel under your abdomen for support, and put a block, pillow or folded towel under your top knee to keep your pelvis in good alignment.

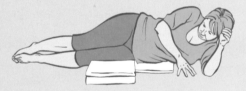

2 ◀ From this side lying position, draw your knees together and start to push up with your right hand. Draw your deep abdominals in smoothly and gently.

3 ▶ Start to press down with your left elbow.

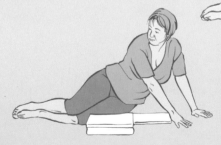

4 ◀ Now use both arms to push yourself up until you are 'side sitting' on your left hip.

5 ▶ Use your hands to adjust your position a little more, as you bring your legs closer into the body.

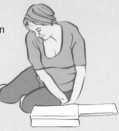

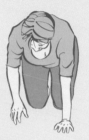

6 ◀ Come over onto all fours, then walk your hands up your thighs to an upright kneeling position.

7 ▶ Then bring your right knee forward and place your right foot ahead of the knee on the mat in front of you.

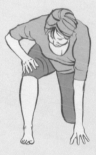

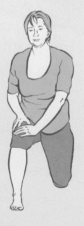

8 ◀ Bring both hands to the right thigh, ready to press them onto the thigh as you breathe out, to bring yourself to standing.

TIP After your baby is born, when bending forwards for nappy-changing tighten your abdomen to prevent it from hanging down, and use your abdominal muscles for support every time you bend.

❶ Shoulder mobility

Improves shoulder mobility • Eases tension in the upper back • Helps strengthen muscles around the upper back • Improves upper back posture

Shoulder rolls

1 Sit on a block, folded towel or straight on the mat, with your legs crossed or out in front of you – whichever is more comfortable. Keep your arms relaxed at your sides. Feel long and lifted through the spine, and ensure that your body weight feels balanced across the left and right sit bones. Make sure that your shoulders are even and released.

2 Breathe in. As you breathe out, draw your shoulders up, over the top and down your back, releasing them down, away from your ears.

Repeat three to five times.

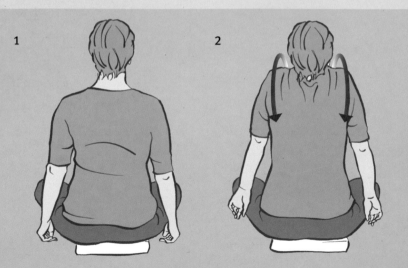

Shoulder blade placement

Sit on a block, folded towel or on the mat, with your legs crossed or out in front of you – whichever is more comfortable. Feel long through the spine and let your hands come up level with your shoulders, arms out in front. Feel your shoulder blades relaxed and flat on your back.

Breathe in and separate your shoulder blades, stretching your fingers further forward, towards the wall opposite you. As you breathe out, draw your side and back ribs down to bring the shoulders flat on your back once again, sliding them down the spine a little. Feel your shoulder blades slide down your back, and the muscles in the middle back sliding down, too. Maintain the long and lifted feeling through the spine throughout.

Repeat three to five times.

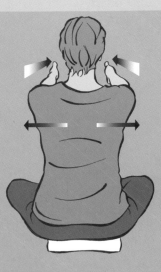

❷ Cat arch

Maintains and increases spinal flexibility • Relieves tense muscles •
Maintains abdominal muscle strength by resisting gravity-pull on all fours

**Caution: If you experience any pain in the lower back or knees, try the
alternative position shown opposite.**

1 Kneel upright with your hands resting on the stability ball about 15 cm
   (6 in) in front of you.

2 Breathe in to prepare and, as you breathe out, allow your body to
   come forward to form a right angle with your legs, as you roll the ball
   out just over half a metre or so (about 2 ft) from you, using your hands

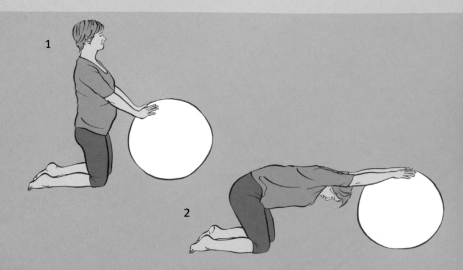

to support yourself outstretched on the ball. Breathe in to stay and enjoy the stretch, feeling your upper back flattening between your arms.

3 Breathe out and, using all your abdominal muscles, start to curl the lower back upwards, tucking under with the tailbone, and draw yourself back through each vertebra in turn, drawing the ball back to the start position.

Repeat five to eight times.

TIP Feel all the abdominal muscles working throughout to support the lower back. Imagine you are gently hugging your baby back towards the pelvis, using your deep abdominal muscles to make the hug.

3

ALTERNATIVE
Cat arch can also be done on all fours, as in the FIRST TRIMESTER sequence (see page 20). Try it this way if you find it more comfortable.

❸ Leg pull

Works the calf muscle, thus helping to reduce swollen ankles by increasing muscle action and blood flow through the leg • Helps stabilize the shoulder blades • Being on all fours helps the baby come into an optimal position for birth

Caution: Stop if your calves begin to cramp.

Kneel on all fours, with your hands under your shoulders and your knees under your hips.

1 Stretch your right leg out behind you, tucking under with the ball of the foot.

1

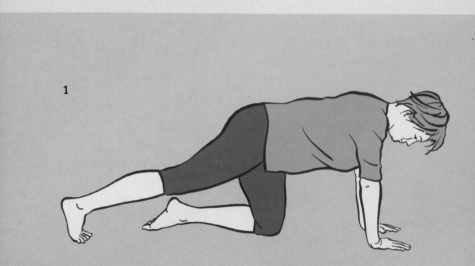

2 Breathe in to prepare and, as you breathe out, rock backwards, pushing your heel further away behind you. Breathe in and release back to the start position.

Repeat five to eight times, rocking over the ball of the foot, pointing and flexing the ankle, and then repeat with the left leg.

TIP Feel the abdominal muscles hugging your baby closer to you, and feel the shoulder blades slide towards your waist as you rock back.

2

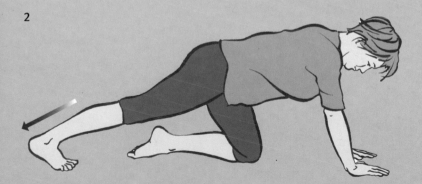

❹ Swimming

Strengthens back muscles • Helps stabilize shoulder blades • Works the buttock muscles

Place a block on its side on the mat (or use something else of a similar shape). This is to give you a guideline for the middle of your body, as you extend your arm and leg during the exercise.

1 Kneel on all fours over the top of the block, with your hands under your shoulders and your knees under your hips. Feel the deep abdominals working to keep your lower back from dipping at the waist.

2 Breathe in to prepare and, as you breathe out, slide your right hand away in front of you, so that your arm comes up in line with your right shoulder. Breathe in to bring the arm back to the start position.

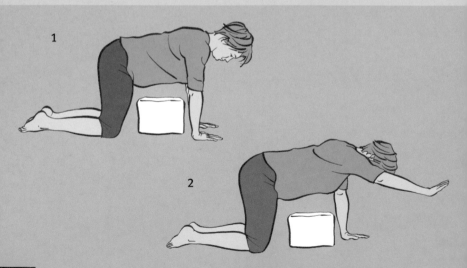

Repeat with the left arm. Continue at this level, if you prefer, repeating five to eight times with each arm. Alternatively, move on to the next step:

3 Breathe in to prepare to slide your right arm away again, but this time, as you breathe out, extend your left leg at the same time as your right arm. Stretch your leg away behind you, bringing it up to hip level if possible, keeping the lower back level and supported using the abdominal muscles. Breathe in to return to the start position, then repeat with your left arm and right leg.

Repeat five to eight times with alternate arms and legs.

TIP Try to keep the mid-line of the body in line with the block. Imagine you are hugging your baby into your pelvis using your deep abdominals. Keep both hip bones facing the floor throughout.

3

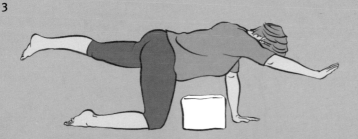

❺ Knee raise

Strengthens buttock muscles (particularly outer part of buttock) • Helps prevent pregnancy 'waddle' when walking

Lie on your left side, with a folded towel and/or block under your head if you wish. Bring your legs together, bending at the knees, and bring your heels in line with your tailbone. Your hips, knees and feet should be 'stacked' one on top of the other.

1 Feel the deep transversus muscle working smoothly and gently, keeping the baby hugged into your pelvis. (The deep abdominals need to work – and keep working – to keep the pelvis still during this exercise.)

1

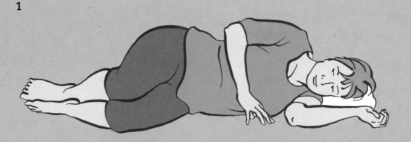

2 Breathe in to prepare and, keeping your feet together, breathe out as you lift your right knee up just as far as you can. Keep your hips stacked one on top of the other and your deep transversus drawn in. Breathe in to return to the start position.

Repeat five to eight times. By the third repetition the outer buttock should begin to feel worked.

Carefully turn over to lie on your right side, and repeat five to eight times with your left knee, to work the left buttock.

TIP Make sure the top hip stays stacked and doesn't roll backwards as you raise your knee.

2

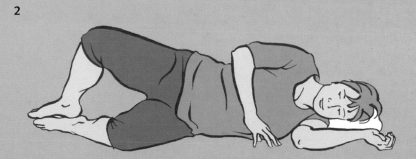

❻ Arm and shoulder opener

Maintains good posture • Opens and stretches front of shoulders •
Helps keep upper back strong • Works the abdominal muscles

Caution: If you feel pain in your lower back, reduce the arm range.

Take your flexi-band and sit on the stability ball, with your sit bones right
on top of the ball, and your spine long and lifted.

1 Hold the flexi-band loosely at either end, with your arms outstretched.

1

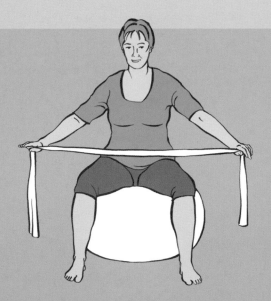

2 Breathe in and lift the band above head level. As you breathe out, bring your arms back down to the start position. Feel the side and back ribs drawing your arms and shoulders down.

Repeat three to five times. You can build up to eight repetitions, if all is working well.

TIP Keep the deep abdominals working to help you stay sitting tall and to support your lower back (and prevent it from over-arching) in this position.

2

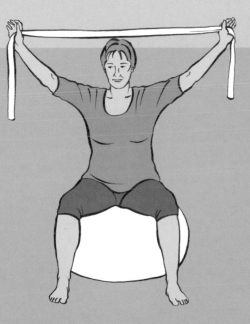

❼ Thigh and buttock strengthener

Maintains and improves thigh strength, ready for an active labour

1   Stand with your back to a wall, with the stability ball at your lower back. Feel your pelvis in neutral and your abdominals drawing in. Walk your feet out two paces from the wall, feet hip-width apart, so that when you bend your knees to 90 degrees they are above your ankles.

2   Breathe in to prepare and, as you breathe out, bend your knees (no more than 90 degrees) and allow the ball to roll up your back. Lean into the ball, keeping your back and pelvis still and your legs parallel. Breathe in to maintain, then breathe out to straighten your knees, pressing through the heels and buttocks to return to the start position.

Repeat ten to twenty *slow* repetitions.

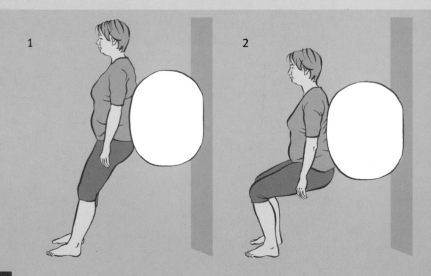

⑧ Wall press-ups

Maintains and improves arm and chest strength, ready for caring for baby

1 Stand facing a wall, feet hip-width apart, keeping the spine in neutral alignment. Step back two paces and lean on the wall, with your hands positioned wider than your shoulders at shoulder height, and your fingers pointing upwards. Try to keep your elbows soft.

2 Breathe in as you bend your elbows, allowing your upper body closer to the wall, keeping your spine in neutral and sliding your shoulder blades down your back. Make sure your elbows are in line with your wrists. Breathe out to push away from the wall, pressing through the arms, and return to the start position. Keep the abdominals working.

Repeat eight to ten times, but try to build up to twenty repetitions.

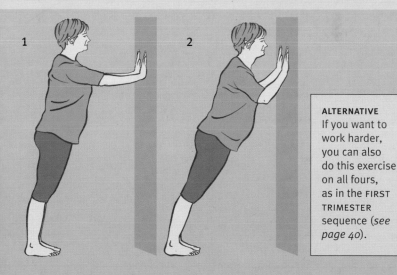

1

2

ALTERNATIVE
If you want to work harder, you can also do this exercise on all fours, as in the FIRST TRIMESTER sequence (*see page 40*).

❾ Major muscle stretches

Gentle stretching helps ease muscle tension and maintain flexibility, especially in the inner thigh and hip flexor, which tighten during pregnancy

Standing calf muscle stretch Stand with your feet hip-width apart and your hands on the wall, shoulder-width apart, and take your right leg out behind you. Allow the heel to gently come down to the mat until you feel a good-quality calf muscle stretch. Hold for eight to ten seconds and repeat with the left leg. Keep breathing as you stretch.

Hip flexor stretch Kneel down and take your right leg out behind you, bringing your left leg up in front so that the foot is well ahead of the knee. Supporting your body weight on your hands, slide your right foot back until you feel a stretch in the right hip. Hold for eight to ten seconds, relax and release, then repeat on the other side.

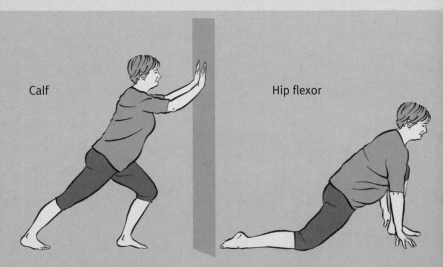

Calf

Hip flexor

Inner thigh stretch Sit on a block, folded towel or on the mat, and allow the soles of your feet to come together. Place your hands just behind you, to help keep the spine long and lifted. Gently ease your knees down until you feel a stretch on the inner thigh. Hold for eight to ten seconds. Maintain easy breathing throughout.

Buttock stretch Sit on a block, folded towel or on the mat, and stretch your left leg out in front of you. Place your right leg across the left, with the sole of the right foot flat on the mat. Now bring your left elbow in front of the right knee and use it to gently draw the right knee across a little. Lift long through the spine until you can feel your right buttock stretching. Repeat on the other side, maintaining easy breathing throughout.

Caution: Do not over-stretch muscles during pregnancy, as the hormone relaxin is already loosening ligaments in preparation for the birth.

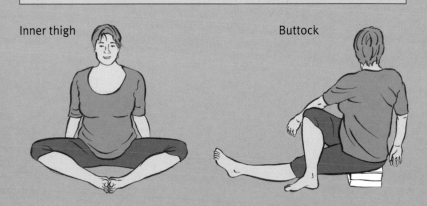

Inner thigh

Buttock

⑩ Relax and stretch

Relaxing lying in a modified shell position or on your side can be really therapeutic during the second trimester. Allow yourself 10 to 15 minutes each day, and you'll find that your energy levels really benefit. Learning to listen to your body and 'turn off' will help during labour, too.

Find a comfortable position, perhaps using a semi-deflated stability ball to relax over. Provided your knees are comfortable, allow your upper body to relax over the ball. Wriggle around until you're comfortable.

You might like to ask a friend with a soothing voice to record the following relaxation script. Play it whenever you want to 'turn off' and relax.

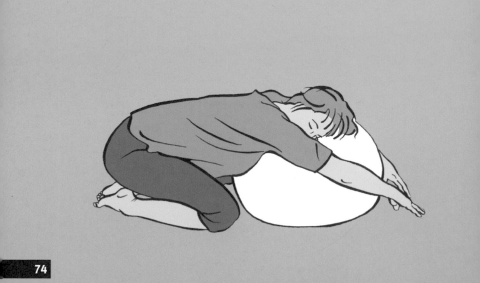

Listen in to your breathing. Taking a long, slow out-breath, just let the in-breath take care of itself. With each out-breath allow your body to sink into your support a little more. Now start to focus on your face. Begin to release tension from the facial muscles. Allow the space between your eyebrows to get a little wider ... the skin across your cheekbones to slide out towards your ears ... your tongue to rest low in your mouth and your lips to be gently parted. Notice the thoughts that will still come into your mind, but send them away for now; you will deal with them later.

Stay for as long as you can, then begin to bring yourself back by increasing your breathing rate. Wriggle your fingers and toes for a minute, visualizing the blood flowing round your body, preparing your body for movement once more. Come up slowly and in your own time.

ALTERNATIVE
If you find it more comfortable, try this relax-and-stretch exercise without the stability ball, or lie on your side, as in the THIRD TRIMESTER sequence (*see page 89*).

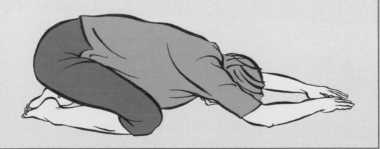

third trimester

This exercise sequence is designed for months seven to nine of your pregnancy. For a slightly longer practice session, you can join the second and third trimester sequences together, though as your pregnancy nears full term and you tire more quickly you may wish to stick to the third trimester only.

Always stop an exercise immediately if you feel any pain (stop and rest, and/or skip the exercise and move on to the next one), and be sure to note any specific cautions that are listed.

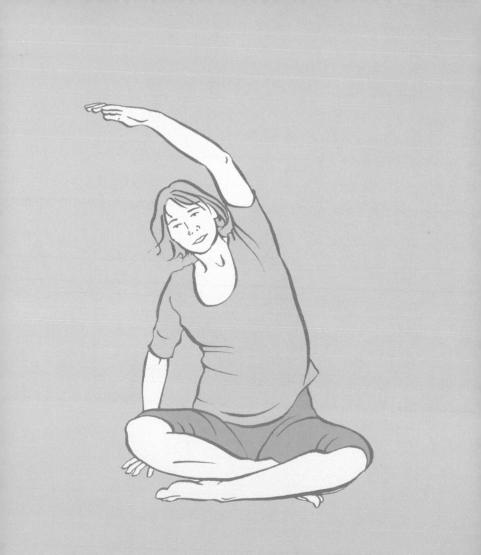

❶ Shoulder mobility

Helps reduce tension in the upper back (which tends to become quite fixed during late pregnancy) • Keeps the upper body flexible and relaxed

Shoulder rolls

Sit on a block, folded towel or straight on the mat, with your legs crossed or out in front of you – whichever is more comfortable. Keep your arms relaxed by your sides. Feel long and lifted through the spine and ensure that your body weight is balanced across your sit bones. Make sure that your shoulders are even and released.

Breathe in. As you breathe out, draw your shoulders up, over the top and down your back, releasing them down, away from your ears.

Repeat three to five times.

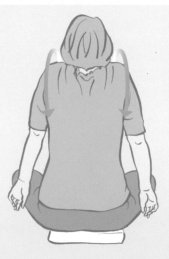

Shoulder blade placement

Sit on a block, folded towel or on the mat with your legs crossed or out in front of you – whichever is more comfortable. Feel long through the spine and let your hands come up level with your shoulders. Feel your shoulder blades relaxed and flat on your back.

Breathe in and separate your shoulder blades, stretching your fingers further forward, towards the wall opposite you. As you breathe out, feel your under-arm and side ribs sink down to draw the shoulder blades back into their normal position. Keep long and lifted through the spine throughout.

Repeat three to five times.

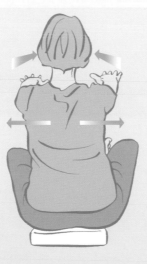

② Cat arch

Helps maintain spinal mobility • Releases tension in the upper and lower back • Kneeling on all fours helps the baby come into an optimal position for birth

Caution: If you experience any pain in your wrists, try this exercise with a stability ball, as used in the second trimester (*see page 60*).

1 Kneel on all fours, with your hands under your shoulders and knees under your hips. Maintain muscle tone in the abdominals to support the lower back, so that your back resembles a table top at the start and finish of the exercise.

1

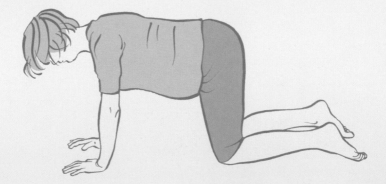

2 Breathe in to prepare and, as you breathe out, draw in the deep abdominals, and start to tuck under with your tailbone, coming up sequentially through each vertebra until your back is arched (like a cat when it stretches). Finally, feel your neck release, allowing you to look through to your knees.

Breathe in to maintain, trying to spread your breath into the side and back of the ribs, and, as you breathe out, bring your pelvis back to normal position, then release through each vertebra in turn, bringing your head back in line with your spine to finish.

Repeat three to five times.

TIP Take care not to let your lower back droop as you return; imagine you are hugging your baby in towards you as you do the exercise.

2

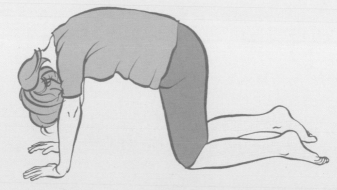

❸ Spinal rotation

Maintains spinal rotation • Releases tension in the upper back and shoulders • Kneeling on all fours helps the baby come into an optimal position for birth

Caution: Avoid twisting the pelvis.

Kneel on all fours with your hands under your shoulders and your knees under your hips, feet relaxed and hip-width apart.

1 Turn your right palm upwards so that the back of your hand is on the mat, and bring your arm back slightly so that your hand is positioned under your chest.

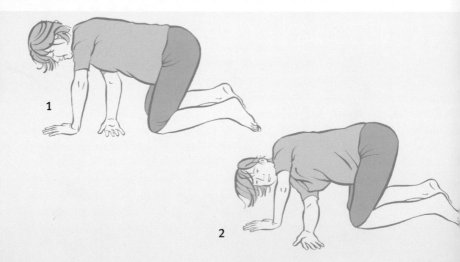

2 Breathe in to prepare and, as you breathe out, allow your right hand to slide across the mat under you, and out beyond your left side, keeping your weight mainly on the left hand and both knees. Breathe in to return to the start position.

Repeat five to eight times, then change hands so that the back of your left hand is on the mat, and repeat five to eight times on the other side.

TIP Keep the abdominal muscles working throughout. You should feel a lovely stretch at the back of the shoulder. Feel the rotation in the upper back, not the knees and/or hips.

ALTERNATIVE
Use a small ball under the back of your hand to allow your arm and body to flow into the position more easily.

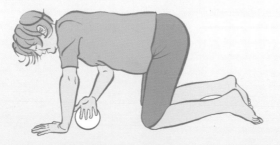

❹ Side stretch

Maintains flexibility in the spine • Lovely stretch for the side of the body, especially in later pregnancy

Caution: If you experience any pain in the lower back, reduce the range of the stretch but keep the spine long and lifted.

Sit on a block, folded towel or directly on the mat, either cross-legged or with your legs out in front of you – whichever is more comfortable.

1 Place your right hand on the mat and lift your left hand up to the ceiling, keeping your shoulders relaxed.

1

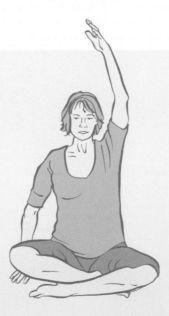

2 Breathe in to prepare and, as you breathe out, stretch your left arm up and over your head to give you a long stretch down the left side of your body. Use your right hand against the mat to support yourself, and keep both buttocks and sit bones on the mat.

Breathe in to draw in the deep transversus smoothly and gently, and bring the body back to the start position.

Repeat two to three times, then repeat on the right side.

2

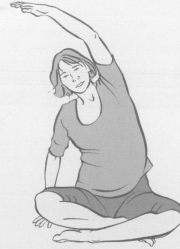

⑤ Shoulder release and arm circle

Maintains good upper back posture • Maintains flexibility in the front of shoulder • Gives a lovely feeling of tension release and relaxation

Caution: If you feel any shoulder pain, start the circle higher up above you.

Shoulder release
Lie on your left side with your head on a folded towel or block and your legs in a side-lying 'table top'. You can also place a folded towel under your baby bump for comfort. Stretch your arms out in front, with a small ball under your right hand. Imagine your right elbow is in a straight plaster cast, so it cannot bend. Keeping the elbow straight, breathe out as you let your right palm roll over the ball, just as far as feels comfortable. Breathe in to roll back, keeping your shoulder blades low. Repeat five to eight times.

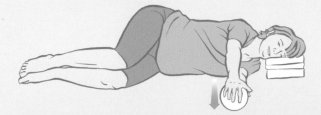

Arm circle

1 Staying on your left side, pick up the ball in your right hand and start to bring it round past your right ear.

2 Continue taking the ball round behind you, as you circle your arm and the ball round past your right hip, to complete the circle.

Repeat five to eight times.

Carefully turn over, and repeat both exercises on the other side, using the left arm to roll and then circle.

TIP Breathe in as you bring the ball past your ear, and breathe out as you bring it past your hip. Keep your hips stacked and avoid rolling back as the arm opens behind. Your breath – and the movement – should remain steady and slow throughout.

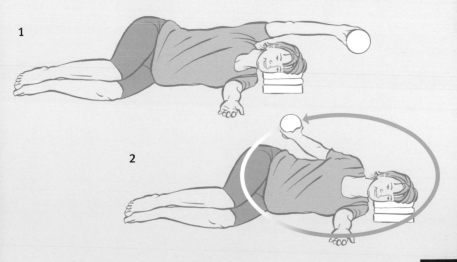

⑥ Hamstring stretch

Maintains the length of the hamstring • Helps keep the pelvis in optimal position • Helps pump blood round the body and prevent swollen ankles

Sit on a block, folded towel or the mat, stretching your left leg out in front of you, with your right leg bent out to the side, in a comfortable position. Use your hands behind you to help lift the spine up and forward, until you get a stretch down the back of the left leg from the sit bone to the back of the knee. Hold for eight to ten seconds, then point the toe and release, and circle the ankle three to five times.

Repeat with the right leg.

TIP To get a good-quality stretch for the hamstring, the knee needs to be straight. Keep your breathing flowing easily as you stretch.

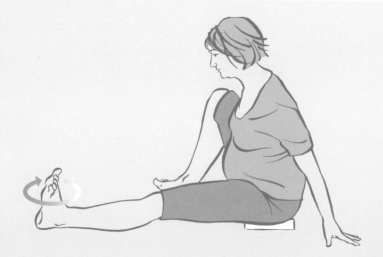

⑦ Relax

Relaxation will help to restore your energy levels and give vital organs a chance to refresh and renew.

Lie on your side, using folded towels or blocks for support. Wriggle around until you feel right. You may like to keep snug and warm under a blanket. Allow a long, slow out-breath and just let your in-breath take care of itself. Use the relaxation for the second trimester (*see page 74*) or, alternatively, think of a place that feels good to be in. It can be anywhere – a field full of wild flowers ... near the sound of splashing water ... a majestic mountain landscape ... Wherever you decide to be, stay there a little longer.

When the time feels right, start to bring yourself back, just as you did in the second trimester. There's no hurry. Take some stretches and then come up through the safe transition sequence shown on pages 56–7.

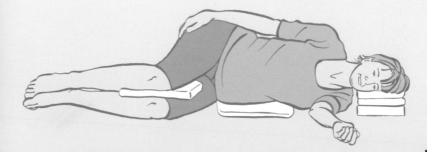

early days

This postnatal exercise sequence is designed to take you from birth up to approximately eight weeks post-birth. Do not move on to the EIGHT WEEKS PLUS *section until you have had your postnatal check-up with your doctor or healthcare professional.*

Always stop an exercise immediately if you feel any pain (stop and rest, and/or skip the exercise and move on to the next one), and be sure to note any specific cautions that are listed.

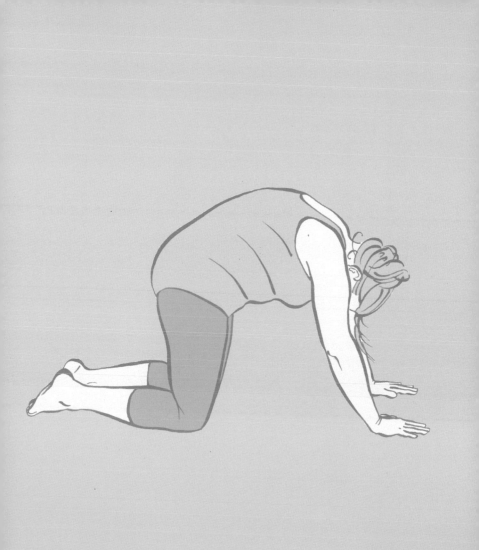

Lifting the baby

During the early postnatal days, your body is gradually recovering from the pregnancy and birth. Even though the baby has been born, however, your body is still susceptible to the loosening effects of the hormone relaxin on the ligaments and joints (as well as being affected by any birth procedures that may have occurred), so great care must still be taken.

New mothers are often advised not to lift and carry heavy items. Easier said than done! If you have lifted a baby's car seat recently – even without the baby in it – you will understand. Get someone else to lift these items for you, if at all possible, during the crucial first ten to fourteen days – especially if your baby's birth involved a Caesarean section, in which case it's essential to give your body a chance to heal itself.

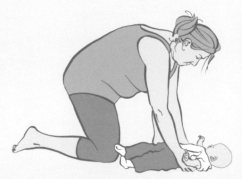

1 ◄ Use a wide base for your feet and keep your spine in neutral. Bend down to kneel on your right knee, keeping your left foot flat on the floor (or vice versa, if you prefer). Kneel close to your baby and place your hands firmly under each side of the body (for newborn babies, scoop one hand underneath the baby's body and the other behind the neck/head for support). Draw in your deep abdominals smoothly and gently.

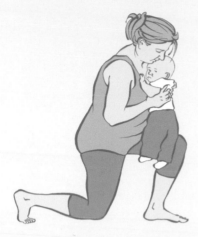

2 ◄ Lift your baby in close to your chest. Tuck under with your right toes and use the strength of your legs to lift you. Feel your leg muscles working strongly to push through the feet and thighs to come up.

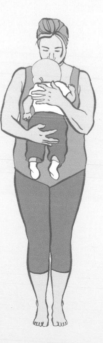

3 ► Once you are upright, continue to hold your baby close into your body to help reduce backache. Consider using a well-fitting baby carrier to keep your baby close.

TIP Draw in the deep abdominals and activate the pelvic floor before any movement, especially if you are carrying your baby.

❶ Pelvic floor

Helps pelvic floor muscles regain strength after being stretched during birth • Helps prevent prolapse of the womb • Strengthens bladder control

Caution: Do not start doing these exercises until you can pass urine normally.

Slow twitch muscles

It's now time to determine your new 'starting block' (*see also pages 11–12*). Sit or stand on a firm surface in good posture, knees slightly apart.

• Tighten your pelvic floor muscles smoothly and gently. Hold for as long as you can, making sure you have something left to release at the end of the hold. Relax the contraction and rest for four seconds. How long could you hold the contraction for? Note this down.

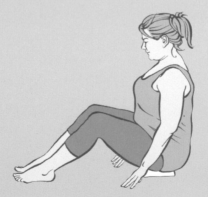

• Repeat the muscle contraction gently and smoothly. Tighten, hold for the number of seconds just noted, and relax, repeating this as many times as you can (up to ten repetitions). Note down the number of repetitions.

You now have your new starting block: the number of seconds you can hold and how many repetitions (up to ten) you can do.

Fast twitch muscles
In the early days these muscles will be considerably weakened, so you'll need to help them become strong again to enable them to react quickly. How many quick and strong contractions can you do? Note down the number, and aim to make the last contraction as strong as the first.

Repeat a balance of the slow and fast twitch muscle contractions three to six times a day.

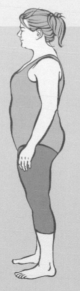

TIP
Like all muscles, the pelvic floor muscles will only get stronger by using them! Try and make these exercises a habit for life – perhaps do them whenever you wash your hands, or make a cup of tea.

❷ Shoulder rolls

Releases shoulder tension, which helps the body cope better in general (shoulder tension tends to significantly increase with the responsibilites a new baby brings)

Caution: If sitting is uncomfortable, consider hiring a 'Valley Cushion' or postnatal cushion to help you sit comfortably during the early postnatal period. Contact your doctor or local birth organization for more details.

Sit on a block, folded towel or mat (or on a special cushion; see above), with your legs crossed or bent out in front of you – whichever is more comfortable.

1   Feel the spine long and lifted, with your shoulders relaxed.

1

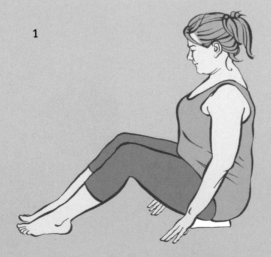

2 Breathe in. As you breathe out, draw your shoulders up, over the top and down your back, releasing them down, away from your ears.

Repeat three to five times.

TIP Try to do this exercise every time you sit down in a regular chair and before and after you feed your baby, to keep your shoulders released and relaxed.

2

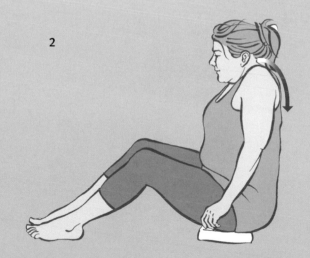

❸ Leg-slide hip release

Helps strengthen the abdominals • Maintains hip-joint flexibility

Caution: Not suitable for the second and third trimesters. If you experience any pain in your lower back, draw your legs in and hug round the back of the thighs to stretch the lower back (*see shell stretch alternative 1, page 107*).

1 Lie on your back with your spine in neutral, with your legs bent and feet flat on the floor. Keep your shoulders relaxed, arms by your sides.

2 As you breathe in, allow your left knee to relax out to the side. Make sure your abdominals stay engaged, so that your right hip doesn't lift.

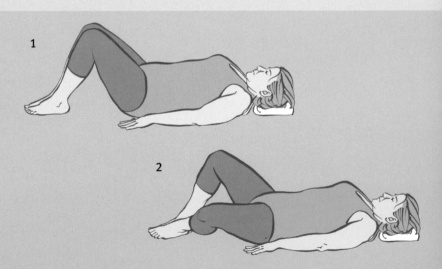

3 Breathe out and slide your left leg down the mat, keeping your foot pointing outwards.

4 Breathe in as you stretch long through the leg, then turn your toes and knee back towards the ceiling. Breathe out and slide the left leg back to the start position, without letting your lower back arch.

Repeat five to eight times, and then repeat with the right leg.

TIP It's important to keep the deep abdominals working smoothly and gently throughout, so that the muscles can gradually strengthen following the pregnancy. Keeping the pelvis level across the body and the spine in neutral is crucial to this exercise. Put your fingertips on your hip bones to check your pelvis doesn't move.

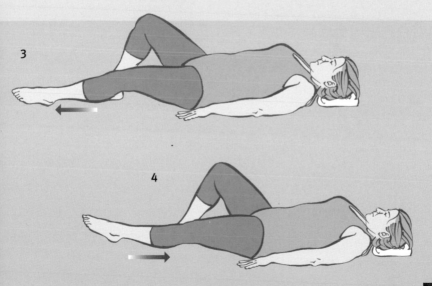

❹ Shoulder release and arm circle

Maintains good upper back posture • Maintains flexibility in the front of shoulder • Gives a lovely feeling of tension release and relaxation

Caution: If you feel any shoulder pain, start the circle higher up above you.

Shoulder release
Lie on your left side with your head on a folded towel or block and your legs in a side-lying 'table top'. Stretch your arms out in front, with a small ball under your right hand. Imagine your right elbow is in a straight plaster cast, so it cannot bend. Keeping the elbow straight, breathe out as you let your right palm roll over the ball, just as far as feels comfortable. Breathe in to roll back, keeping your shoulder blades low. Repeat five to eight times.

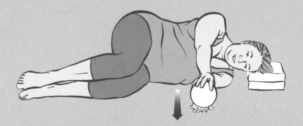

Arm circle

1 Staying on your left side, pick up the ball in your right hand and start to bring it round past your right ear.

2 Continue taking the ball round behind you, as you circle your arm and the ball round past your right hip, to complete the circle.

Repeat five to eight times.

Carefully turn over, and repeat both exercises on the other side, using the left arm to roll and then circle.

TIP Breathe in as you bring the ball past your ear, and breathe out as you bring it past your hip. Keep your hips stacked and avoid rolling back as the arm opens behind. Your breath – and the movement – should remain steady and slow throughout.

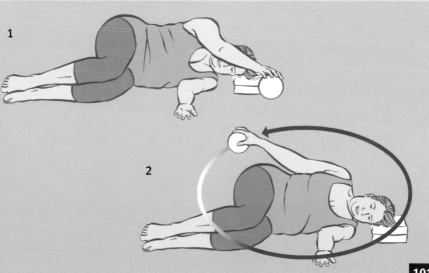

⑤ Cat arch

Improves and maintains abdominal group of muscles • Helps keep the spine flexible

Caution: If you experience any pain in your wrists, try this exercise with a stability ball, as used in the second trimester (*see page 60*).

1   Kneel on all fours, with your hands under your shoulders and knees under your hips. Keep your whole back in line, like a table top, and the back of your neck long and level with your spine, with your shoulders released down your back. Keep your deep abdominal muscles activated to prevent the lower back from sagging.

1

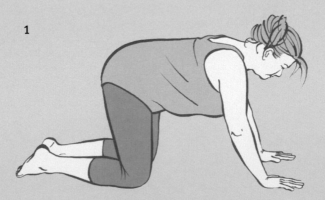

2 Breathe in to prepare and, as you breathe out, draw the abdominal muscles in gently and smoothly, then curl under with your tailbone and start to tighten your abdominal 'zip' muscles (rectus abdominus), lifting your spine up towards the ceiling, each vertebra in turn. Lastly, feel your neck release to allow you to look through to your knees.

Breathe in – into the wide rib cage – to maintain, then, as you breathe out, reverse the exercise, taking care not to let the lower back sag as you return to the start position.

Repeat five to eight times.

TIP Feel the whole abdominal group of muscles initiating the movement and working throughout, and the lower back opening up. Try to keep your shoulder blades released, down the spine.

2

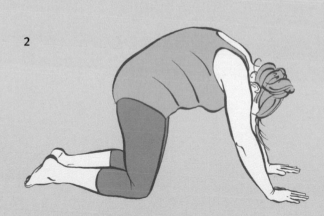

⑥ Hip lifts

Strengthens the buttocks and hamstrings (strengthening the buttock muscles is important for posture, as these muscles weaken and lengthen during pregnancy)

Caution: Not suitable for the second and third trimesters. If you experience any pain in the lower back, try to lengthen your lower back by curling your pubic bone up towards your navel.

1   Lie on your back with your feet and knees hip-width apart, feet flat on the floor. Keep your lower back and pelvis in neutral and feel your shoulder blades soften and flatten down your back. Rest your arms at your sides and relax your hands, elbows and front of shoulders.

1

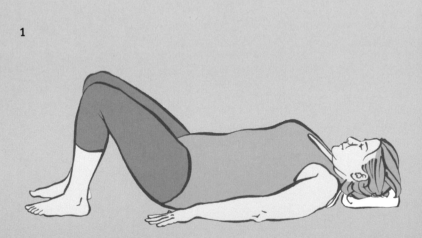

2 Breathe in to prepare and, as you breathe out, squeeze the buttocks and lift the pelvis up without articulating through the spine – as though a crane has lifted it straight up. Your body will then be on a diagonal line through the shoulders, hips and knees. Breathe in to maintain, and then breathe out to bend at the knees and hips, to come back down to the start position.

Repeat five to eight times.

TIP When in the lifted position, feel long through the body, making sure you don't over-lift and cause any discomfort in the lower back. Move your feet closer to your buttocks to support the back.

2

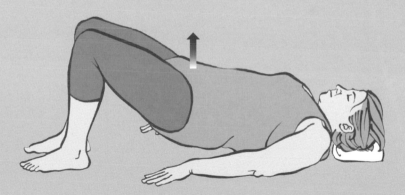

❼ Shell stretch

Lengthens and stretches the lower back, helping to relieve backache
• Works the abdominal and pelvic floor muscles

Caution: If you experience any pain in your knees, try one of the alternative positions shown opposite.

Kneel with your knees slightly apart, then sit on your heels and allow your spine to come forward over your legs. Relax your arms, either out in front of you or alongside your body. You can use pressure on your hands to help the lower back stretch.

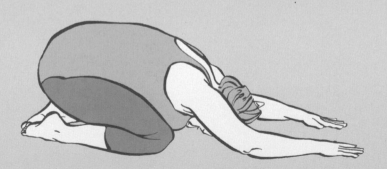

Breathe in to prepare and, as you breathe out – keeping your abdominals deeply drawn in – allow your side and back ribs to expand out, as you continue easy breathing, holding the stretch for eight to ten seconds.

To come out of the stretch, place your hands under your shoulders and uncurl through each vertebra in turn, to return to an upright position. Keep the abdominals engaged throughout.

TIP Feel your lower back open and your tailbone drop down as you stretch. Try to release any tension in the shoulders.

ALTERNATIVE 1
Lie on your back, allow both legs to come into the chest and hug round the back of the thighs. Feel your lower back open and release.

ALTERNATIVE 2
Lie on your back, bring your left leg into the chest and hug round the back of the left thigh. Allow your right leg to go long down the mat. Feel the lower back open slightly and feel the right hip open and release. Repeat with the right leg. Keep breathing throughout.

eight weeks plus

This postnatal exercise sequence is designed to take you from eight weeks post-birth onwards, up to about five months after the birth. Do not attempt these exercises until you have had your postnatal check-up with your doctor or healthcare professional. For a full postnatal workout, you can join both postnatal exercise routines together.

Always stop an exercise immediately if you feel any pain (stop and rest, and/or skip the exercise and move on to the next one), and be sure to note any specific cautions that are listed.

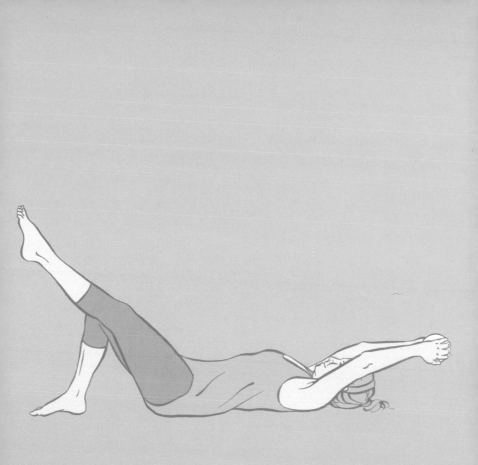

❶ Pelvic tilt

Helps shorten the rectus abdominus

Caution: Not suitable for later pregnancy. If you find that your abdomen pushes up to a ridge down the centre as you perform this exercise, find a local postnatal-exercise specialist to help you get the exercise correct.

Lie on your back with your knees bent and feet flat on the floor, hip-width apart, with your spine and pelvis in neutral alignment. Keep your arms relaxed at your sides.

1   Breathe in to prepare and, as you breathe out, start to tilt the pelvis by drawing your ribs down towards your hips and your hips up towards your ribs. Feel the rectus abdominus creating the movement.

1

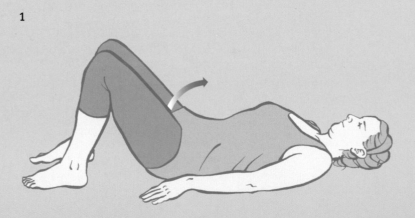

The pubic bone will lift only a little. Feel your lower back pressing lightly into the mat.

2   Breathe in to maintain, and then breathe out to return the spine to neutral again.

You can build up your strength by staying in the tilt for several in- and out-breaths, before returning to neutral.

Repeat five to eight times.

TIP Feel your abdomen scooping in towards the spine, and focus on drawing the pubic bone and waist closer together. Keep the buttocks and shoulders relaxed throughout.

2

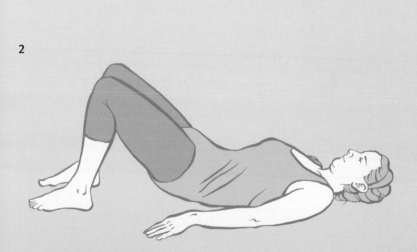

❷ Hip rolls

Strengthens the abdominals (particularly rectus abdominus) • Works the buttocks and hamstrings • Improves spinal mobility

Caution: Not suitable for the second and third trimesters.

Lie on your back with your knees bent and feet flat on the floor, hip-width apart, and your spine and pelvis in neutral alignment. Keep your arms relaxed at your sides.

1   Breathe in to prepare and, as you breathe out, draw your ribs down towards your hips and your hips up towards your ribs, imprinting the spine. Feel your lower back pressing lightly into the floor. Breathe in to maintain and, as you breathe out again, start to lift your tailbone off

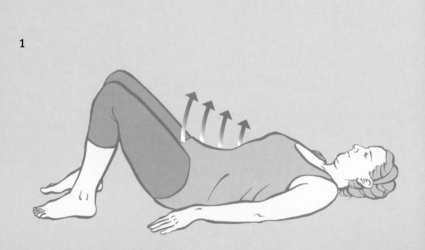

1

the floor and then peel your spine up, vertebra by vertebra, breathing out all the way until your knees, hips and shoulders form a diagonal line.

2 Breathe in to maintain, keeping the buttocks activated – without lifting any higher – and feel long through the diagonal line. Then breathe out to reverse the movement, bringing the spine back down, vertebra by vertebra, feeling the ribs draw down towards the hips, opening the lower back. Last of all, release the pelvis into neutral by bringing your tailbone back to the floor.

Repeat five to eight times.

TIP Try to scoop the abdominal muscles in, to help the mobility of the spine, and make sure you breathe out as you move, both when coming up and going down.

2

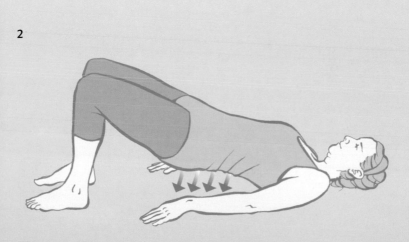

❸ Side leg lift

Improves and maintains buttock strength

Lie on your left side with your body and legs in line, and your shoulders and hips each 'stacked' one above the other. Bend your left (lower) ankle to help you balance, and place your right (upper) hand on the mat in front of your body, to help stabilize you. You can place a folded towel between your head and arm to make your neck more comfortable, if you wish.

1 As you breathe in, draw in your abdominal muscles smoothly, then point your toes and lift your upper leg to hip height only, keeping the knee facing the front and stretching long through the leg.

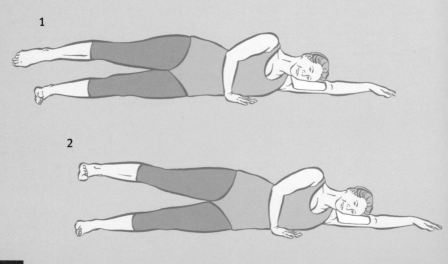

2 Breathe out, flexing the ankle, and feel a strong stretch through your heel as you bring your leg down back to the start position.

Repeat five to eight times, then carefully roll over onto your right side, and repeat with the left leg (*see also advanced option, below*).

TIP Feel the waist staying long on both sides of the body, and feel stretched through the whole body as you work. Keep the abdominals drawn in smoothly and gently throughout.

ADVANCED To work to the next level, bend the lower leg for stability and draw a small circle from the top hip. Rotate five times in one direction, then five in reverse, and keep breathing as you work. Repeat with the other leg.

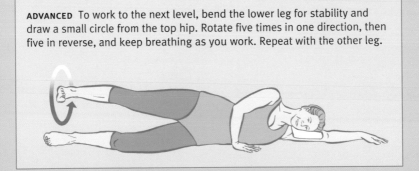

❹ Spinal rotation

Opens the front of the shoulders • Stretches the chest muscles • Increases the mobility of the spine

Caution: If you experience any pain in the lower back, reduce the range of the arm movement.

1 Lie on your left side, with a block or folded towel under your head. Bring your knees up level with your hips (into a side-lying 'table top') and allow both arms to lie out in front of you, keeping your shoulder blades drawn down your back, and your lower back in neutral.

2 Breathe in to bring your right hand up, keeping your shoulders relaxed. Follow your thumbnail with your eyes, so your head turns comfortably.

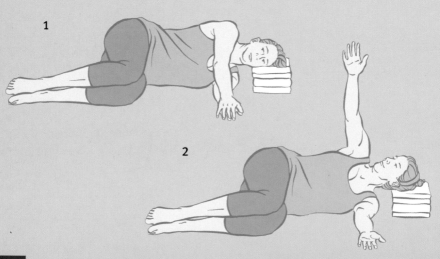

3 As you breathe out, open your right shoulder, taking your hand and arm away behind you, just as far as feels comfortable. Breathe in to maintain, feeling the stretch from one set of fingertips to the other.

Breathe out as you draw in the deep abdominals, feeling your right ribs drawing down towards your pubic bone. Using the strength of the abdominals, bring your right arm back to the start position.

Repeat five to eight times, then carefully turn over to repeat the spinal rotation on the other side.

TIP Keep your knees heavy and together throughout. Feel space between your ears and shoulders, and feel the abdominals initiating the movement, particularly as you return.

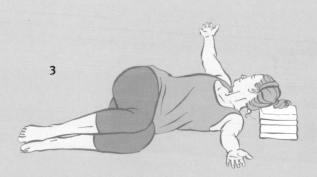

3

⑤ Single-leg stretch

Strengthens the abdominal muscles

Caution: Not suitable for the second and third trimesters.

Lie on your back with your knees bent and feet flat on the floor, then raise your left leg up into 'table top'. Holding a small ball between your hands, bring your hands above your chest, keeping your shoulders relaxed and away from your ears. Begin with your spine in neutral.

1   Breathe in to prepare and, as you breathe out, imprint your spine slightly by drawing your ribs down towards your hips and your hips up towards your ribs. Feel the abdominals flattening and drawing in.

1

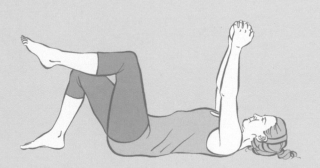

2 Breathe in once more, then, as you breathe out, allow your left leg to stretch long, keeping the left thigh parallel to the right thigh – do not allow it to drop. As you stretch your leg, take your hands – and the ball – over your head, keeping the imprint with your spine to prevent your back from arching. Breathe in to return to the start position.

Repeat five to eight times, and then repeat with the right leg.

TIP It's vital that your lower back eases into the mat in this exercise (imprinting). This requires a lot of concentration and work for the abdominals, so you can leave your arms by your sides to begin with, if you prefer (*see alternative position, below*).

2

ALTERNATIVE
This exercise can also be done with just the legs, leaving your arms relaxed at your sides.

❻ Upper back strengthener

Strengthens lower and upper back muscles • Works the deep abdominals

Caution: If you experience pain in your lower back or breasts, try and draw in the deep abdominal muscles a little more or adjust your position.

1 Kneel with your body upright, with both hands on the stability ball just in front of you.

2 Keeping your body straight and your hands steadying the ball, lean against the ball, allowing your pubic bone to press against it, then relax your hands lightly on the front of the ball.

3 Allow your body to take the shape of the ball, keeping your arms and hands relaxed, maintaining easy breathing all the while.

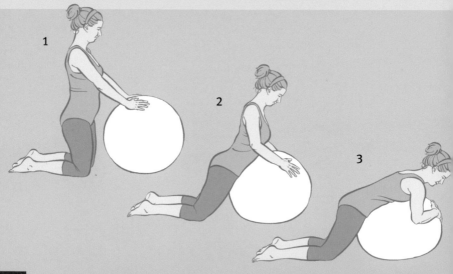

4 Now, breathe in to draw the shoulders down your back, at the same time as drawing in your deep transversus muscle. Breathe out to lift the upper back away from the ball (or mat; *see alternative*). Breathe in to maintain, and then breathe out again to return to the position in step 3.

Keep your head aligned with the upper back, and your buttocks relaxed. Feel long through the top of the ears, and avoid pushing on the ball with your hands.

Repeat five to eight times, then take a shell stretch to finish (*see page 106*).

TIP Feel the upper and lower back muscles working as you lift and lengthen the body away from the ball (or mat). Activate your deep abdominals, drawing them away from the ball as you work. When you breathe in, do so into the side ribs.

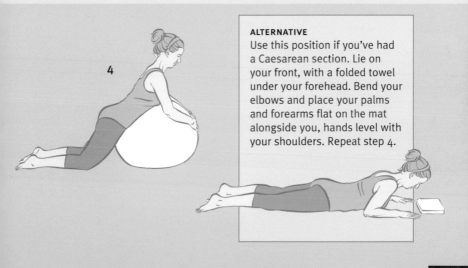

ALTERNATIVE
Use this position if you've had a Caesarean section. Lie on your front, with a folded towel under your forehead. Bend your elbows and place your palms and forearms flat on the mat alongside you, hands level with your shoulders. Repeat step 4.

❼ Pelvic circles

Loosens and eases tension in the lower back

Sit on the stability ball with your feet flat on the floor, roughly hip-width apart. Your hips should be slightly higher than your knees, so that there's a gentle slope down the thighs to the knees. Rest your hands on your thighs or on the ball.

Picture the base of the pelvis as the four points of the compass – north, east, south and west. Visualize the four bones at the base of the pelvis corresponding to the same points. Keeping your spine in neutral, with your back long and lifted and your shoulders relaxed, start to circle round the points of the compass.

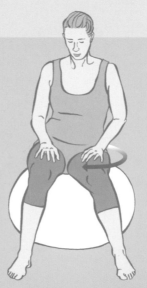

Feel the circle round from north (the pubic bone), to east (the right sit bone), to south (the tailbone), to west (the left sit bone). Then reverse and circle round the other way. Maintain easy breathing throughout.

Repeat three to five times in each direction.

TIP Feel the abdominals lightly working. Keep your chest lifted and your spine long, with your shoulders relaxed, and avoid arching your back excessively as you circle.

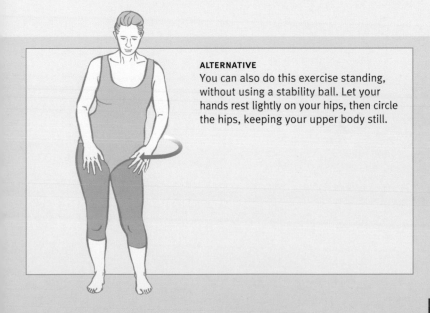

ALTERNATIVE
You can also do this exercise standing, without using a stability ball. Let your hands rest lightly on your hips, then circle the hips, keeping your upper body still.

❽ Adductor stretch

Lengthens the inner thigh muscles

Sit on the mat, or folded towel, with the soles of your feet together, and let your knees open to the sides. Place your fingers on the mat behind you, and keep your spine in neutral. Breathe in to prepare and, as you breathe out, gently ease your knees outwards until you feel a stretch on both inner thighs (the muscles from the groin to the inner side of the knee). Try to draw in the deep abdominals, and keep the spine long and lifted.

Hold for eight to ten seconds, maintaining easy breathing, and release.

You may find it easier to hold your feet and lean forward in order to find this stretch (*see alternative, page 53*). See what works best for you.

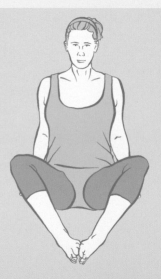

⑨ Buttock stretch

Lengthens the buttock muscles

Sit on the floor with your right leg straight out in front and your left leg bent over your straight leg, with your foot flat on the floor, close to the right knee. Feel long through the spine, as though you are lifting up away from your sit bones. Keep both buttocks on the floor while you draw your left knee across your body with your right hand until you feel a stretch in the left buttock.

Hold for eight to ten seconds, then release and change legs to stretch the other buttock. Maintain easy breathing throughout. (For other suitable stretches see shoulder opener, *page 52*; hip flexor stretch, *page 72*; hamstring stretch, *page 88*; and lower back stretch, *page 107*.)

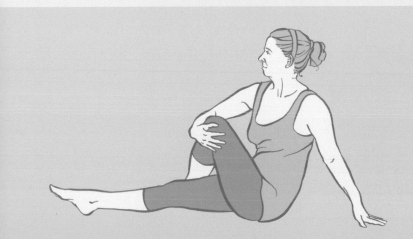

⑩ Pat on the back

Put your left hand on your right shoulder, and your right hand on your left shoulder – and give yourself a big pat on the back! You have now finished the postnatal workout. You've done well, and you need to tell yourself this occasionally!

Give yourself a pat on the back each time you complete the workout.

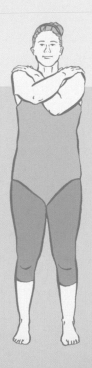

Keep motivated!

Keeping active will make you feel better and healthier, and it also improves your posture – which in turn means your whole body is working more efficiently.

Try to keep practising the postnatal routines and pelvic floor exercises on a regular basis, to help you get back in shape. The routines don't take long, and you'll really feel the difference. Start gently with EARLY DAYS, and then – when you feel ready (and you've had your postnatal check-up with your doctor) – move on to EIGHT WEEKS PLUS, joining both sequences together for a longer workout, if you feel up to it.

You can even set your baby up to watch you while you practise; babies are fascinated by activity, so you can do your exercise and entertain him or her at the same time!

If you can, fit a brisk walk with your baby into your everyday routine. Walk until you feel warmed up. This will help you lose extra fat as well as raising your mood – and it will help your baby to sleep better, too. Why not try alternating your exercise, with Pilates practice one day and a walk the next, so you are doing some form of activity on at least five out of seven days.

Above all, keep it up! Make your Pilates practice a habit for life, and you'll ensure that, once you're back in shape, you *stay* in shape.

> **NOTE** When your monthly periods return, take extra care with body alignment and pay special attention to safe transition movements; research shows that the hormone relaxin is released on days 14 and 26 of the 28-day cycle. This means you may be more prone to muscle injury on these days.

ABOUT THE AUTHOR

Meg Walker has taught postnatal aerobics since 1990, having trained with the YMCA. She added pregnancy exercise to her qualifications in 1994 and has specialized in Pilates for pregnant and postnatal women since 2004. She is a founder member of the Guild of Pregnancy and Postnatal Exercise Instructors, a non-profit organization that provides fitness information for new and expectant mothers, including directory listings to help women find qualified instructors in their local area (visit www.postnatalexercise.co.uk).

Meg's strong conviction that the benefits of exercise aid recovery and adjustment to the stresses and strains of new motherhood has been central to her work over the last twenty years in encouraging mothers to exercise appropriately.

ABOUT THE CONSULTANT

Judy DiFiore is a respected authority on pregnancy and postnatal exercise, and has been teaching exercise for twenty years, specializing in ante- and postnatal exercise for the last fifteen years. Meg trained with Judy when she was a tutor for YMCA Fitness Industry Training. Judy is a tutor for the Guild of Pregnancy and Postnatal Exercise Instructors, and Director of Pushy Mothers Ltd – a UK company offering buggy workouts for new mums. Judy is also the author of the postnatal-exercise bible *The Complete Guide to Postnatal Fitness*, now in its third edition.

ACKNOWLEDGEMENTS

Many thanks to Elaine Partington, Malcolm Smythe and Tessa Monina for their considerable input, and to exercise mothers Rosie, Inger, Jane, Nicky, Gill and baby Finley. Special thanks to Judy DiFiore for her advice and support, and to Samantha Gillard for checking pelvic floor text and Anette Holtmeyer-Cole for her encouragement. Lastly, thanks to my husband Eliot for his practical and loving support and patience.